PMDD and Relationships

PMDD and Relationships

Living on a Prayer
Living with PMDD

Liana Laverentz

PMDD and Relationships

Lily Pond Publications

Cover Art by *Rae Monet, Inc. Design*

Living on a Prayer, Living with PMDD
P.O. Box 196
Harborcreek, PA 16421-0196
www.livingwithpmdd.com

Publishing History
First Edition, July, 2015
Print ISBN 978-1-943734-01-6
Digital ISBN 978-1-943734-00-9

Published in the United States of America

Disclaimer

This book's intention is to inform and educate. It is not to replace medical advice given by your health care professional. It is recommended that you consult your doctor or health professional before following any therapeutic advice, especially if you have a pre-existing medical condition. Never reduce or discontinue your prescribed medication without the consent of your doctor. The author cannot take medical or legal responsibility for illness arising out of the failure to seek medical advice from a doctor or nurse practitioner.

Praise for Living on a Prayer, Living with PMDD

————◆————

I have read so many things on PMDD and nothing has ever been more correct than this... I will be showing this to my boyfriend...Thank you.

～⋎～

I want to thank you from the bottom of my heart for all the information you share. This has helped me get diagnosed and on the right track to self awareness and recovery. I cannot express how much you have helped me.

～⋎～

Thank you so much for your wonderful blogs...I can't wait to go home tonight and talk to my husband and get him to read these comments from other men going through the hell he has endured!

～⋎～

Great help...I needed this so bad because as a man I never understood this because I don't have it but reading this may have just saved my relationship... Thanks.

～⋎～

Thank you so much for this. It so totally spoke to and of me, I could hardly finish the article for the tears in my eyes. Someone understands what I'm living with.

～⋎～

My husband said it's like someone has been living in our house and recording everything we go through.

～⋎～

Dedication

To Mom, who showed me how it's done.
Thank you and I love you.

Table of Contents

Author's Note

PMDD and Relationships is based in part on several blog posts I wrote between May 2010 and May 2015. In this book I have updated the affected blog posts to reflect the most current information available at publication. Other sections of the book are new material, and information provided in them may be repeated in other titles in my PMDD series, the availability of which can be found on my blog or website.

This book is not intended to be read like a novel, rather more like a reference book. Parts of it are addressed to women with PMDD, while other sections would be more beneficial to their partners. I trust you to figure out which is which, and know which chapters you do and do not need to read. If you do read it all the way through, some information may be repeated.

May 2015

A few years ago I read a book by a famous television personality on happiness, or how to be happy. By all accounts, according to that book, I should have been the happiest woman on the planet. In case I might be missing a few opportunities for happiness, it offered seventeen powerful tips for living a happier life. All of which I at the time already practiced regularly, if not daily.

But still, then and now, on some days happiness eludes me. Why is this? Because there are times you simply cannot be happy when you have PMDD, also known as the mood disorder Pre-Menstrual Dysphoric Disorder.

Plain and simple, during an episode of PMDD, nothing makes you happy. No-thing. You can have fleeting moments of joy, but that's all they are. Fleeting.

Let's break it down. PMDD. That first D stands for Dysphoric, the opposite of euphoric. Euphoric means happy, dysphoric means depressed. As in depression. The kind of depression suffered by at least the 164 million people in the United States who were given prescriptions for antidepressants in 2008 alone. No one knows how many more there are, not being treated with drug therapy, talk therapy, or any other kind of therapy. Depression, while not a rich man's disease, can only be diagnosed and treated if you have the means and mindset to see a doctor and pay for the treatment.

But PMDD is different. PMDD is a disorder that comes and goes in concert with a woman's menstrual cycle. Actually, disorder is misleading. PMDD is more than a simple disorder of the mind, as defined by the DSM-V. If left untreated, PMDD can expand in scope from 2-3 days a month to all but 2-3 days a month, or until a woman is left with no "good days" to enjoy.

PMDD can be inherited, and can begin as early as a woman's first period. Mostly, according to medical experts on the subject, the onset arrives in a woman's twenties or thirties, and if left untreated, grows progressively worse until menopause.

As I look back on my life, I can see I was an early starter. I remember an episode in college that kept me in bed for three weeks, feeling listless, hopeless, and lethargic. Then suddenly it disappeared, and I had to work like a maniac to complete all my coursework and pass the semester.

I've often likened my life to that of a salmon swimming upstream. Always behind, always swimming against the tide, never managing to fully get where I am going. For years I thought it was my time-management skills. Now I realize it was the PMDD kicking my butt.

Because when I'm not in the throes of PMDD, I can time manage like nobody's business. I can get more done in a day than four people and get more done in a week than most people can in a month. I've managed projects, contests, social events, PR events, organized banquets, grand openings, conferences, committees, written four books, edited over seventy more, and designed and overseen the building of two houses. I've won awards for most of those things, and have the certificates, plaques, clocks, and trophies to show it.

But when I'm having a PMDD episode, I can barely shower and get dressed. My mind is fuzzy and disoriented, my thoughts scattered, my emotions raw and unstable. I ache all over physically, my brain either feels like it's burning or has an iron band wrapped around it, I feel like I am moving through molasses, and I have absolutely no motivation. I don't want to see anybody, much less talk to them, or do much of anything. My prevailing thought patterns are, "Why bother? Nobody cares anyway. What's the use?" and "Take me now, Lord. Just get it over with and take me. I can't possibly be of any use to anyone in this state."

Oddly enough, even on the worst of my PMDD days, I can rouse myself to help a family member, friend, or even a stranger in need. It's doing the things I need to do for *myself* that get put off until I feel better. Because in my PMDD state I. Just. Don't. Feel. Like. It. Nor do I consider my wants, needs, or desires worth the effort. Every negative thought is magnified until I am practically paralyzed as far as decision making and motivation goes. That includes decisions as simple as what to eat or wear. What if I screw up, make the wrong choice—and I know I will—my PMDD brain is telling me it's inevitable.

But somehow I can shove that all aside when someone truly needs me to be there for them. My guess is it has something to do with the bonding hormone, oxytocin. But I'll talk about that more later on.

Like I said, undiagnosed PMDD can only get worse over time. It can also predispose you toward major depressive episodes, both in response to life stresses and during times when women are most vulnerable to depression, such as post-partum, and peri- and post-menopausal. In 2009 I had an episode that lasted for weeks and weeks and weeks, which set me on the path to starting my blog, *Living on a Prayer, Living with PMDD*, and writing this book.

I now know that back then I was experiencing a low-grade perimenopausal depression that my PMDD exacerbated until it became unbearable. It forced me to take the time out to see to my own health and wellness—to put *me* first.

Why didn't I do something about my PMDD earlier? Well, for the first 25 years, I didn't know PMDD existed. I just thought I had regular PMS, and since 80% of menstruating women experience some symptoms of PMS, I didn't see why I couldn't just deal with it like everyone else. Was I really that incapable of coping with something women deal with every day? My pride refused to allow for that possibility.

Besides, the episodes came and went. And as soon as they went, I was too busy playing catch up to stop and try to figure out what was wrong with me. All I knew was I was free to be myself again, and frankly, for those first 25 years, out of sight was out of mind. I was just grateful to be back on track again.

Until the next time. For years, I consoled myself with the idea that "this too, shall pass," and in a few days it would be over. I could then get on with my life again, as a wife, mother, part-time office worker, and writer. I didn't realize what a huge disservice I was doing to myself, allowing my PMDD to progress. Besides, I still thought it was simple PMS, and all the prevailing medical literature at the time said there was nothing I could do but "live with it." To be sure, there were lifestyle and dietary changes I could make, and off and on I tried. But every effort seemed to fail after a few weeks, and I thought it was due to a lack of willpower.

Wrong. It was the PMDD. PMDD being cyclical as it is, what starts out as a brilliant idea and the willpower and determination behind it, all too soon devolves into a stupid idea with no willpower or motivation to support it. Sometimes this change in perception comes as soon as two weeks after the onset of your period, sometimes you're blessed with a full three weeks before your world view turns upside down again. Your PMDD brain is also a crafty character, and very adaptable to change—or, rather, finding ways to subvert any positive changes you may make.

PMDD is all about self-preservation, believe me. There's nothing your PMDD brain won't do to keep running the show. When women commit suicide to escape their PMDD, chances are they feel it's the only way to shut up the bully in their PMDD brain.

PMDD can strike both around the time of a woman's ovulation, and pre-menstrually. It can also occur post-menstrually in atypical cases—which was what confused me for so many years. It wasn't until 2010 that I learned it could also occur *after* your period begins. Mine comes without fail on the third day of my period—when it chooses to come. It doesn't come every month, and sometimes it comes twice a month, which only adds to the confusion. For years I had only mild symptoms pre-menstrually, mostly food cravings and anger, edginess, and irritation, with my major depressive symptoms coming *after* my period.

All the literature I read said the symptoms of PMDD came only pre-menstrually. So I didn't feel I could qualify for a diagnosis of PMDD. Something else had to be going on with me, in addition to what I thought was ordinary PMS, but it didn't have a name that I could find, and I didn't know how to go about explaining it to anyone. To tell the truth, I just thought I was crazy.

In the past few years, however, my symptoms have been coming pre-menstrually, post-menstrually, and during what I call "special" months, during ovulation. I would barely get over one episode before another began, until early 2009, when I had one that lasted five weeks.

It was after the five-week episode that I knew I had to do something. I couldn't afford to lose weeks of productivity at a time. I knew I wasn't depressed, not in the way of Major Depressive Disorder, because the symptoms came and went. Finally I started charting them, and after two months, per the instructions in all the books I read, I went to my doctor and was diagnosed with PMDD.

That's when the real fun began. Now that my PMDD had been confirmed, it was time to read (and in many cases, re-read) everything I possibly could about it. I had been collecting information about PMS and PMDD for years. Since 1985. But I hadn't looked into it seriously since 1994, when I read *Women's Bodies, Women's Wisdom*, by Dr. Christiane Northrup.

Unfortunately, at the time, in all but a few medical research circles, PMDD was still a faraway blip on the general public's horizon. Most of the information available to the general public at that time was about PMS, with references to PMDD as simply a "more severe" form of PMS—which has since been proven through clinical studies to be untrue.

PMDD is a medical condition separate and apart from PMS. However, since it affects women, and occurs as part of our menstrual cycles, it's still lumped in with PMS and PME or Pre-Menstrual Exacerbation of existing disorders, such as arthritis, asthma, lupus, fibromyalgia, diabetes, or, yes, depression.

Even so, I can't tell you how grateful I was to read that a woman's hormonal cycles are part and parcel of being a woman, that they are natural and normal, and in terms of the mind-body connection, are to be celebrated and honored instead of cursed and ridiculed and swept under the rug.

I wasn't crazy. This really was happening. And there was a medical explanation for it. My body was not working properly during those times of the month. This made me edgy, angry, weepy, sad, muddle-headed and hungry. It was okay. It was normal. It was natural. All I had to do was watch my diet, take vitamins, exercise, maintain a healthy weight, listen to the wisdom of my body, rest when I could, and grin and bear it when I couldn't.

So I did—until, like I said, the episodes started lasting eight to ten days, and then weeks at a time. Until I discovered the latest research on PMDD, produced in the past decade, which states that no matter what you do, as long as your *brain* does not work properly, no amount of healthy eating, exercise, vitamins or herbs, meditation exercises, motivational books and CDs, self-talk, psychological counseling, or acts of goodwill will eliminate your PMDD.

All of the above will no doubt make you healthier overall, and may make you feel better more days than not, but they will *not* make your PMDD go away.

Not by themselves, that is.

Knowledge is power, and with the information included in this book, you will have the basic tools needed to create better relationships throughout your life, and to come to understand and deal with *your* PMDD (or that of your loved one) at *your* speed and level.

Be well. You deserve no less.

Introduction

———◆———

Creating my Living With PMDD Blog

Living With PMDD Blog

Hi, I'm Liana, and for the past 40+ years I've had PMDD. The first 25 years I had no idea what was going on inside me, and I simply thought I was crazy. Not wanting anyone else to know that, I kept it to myself. For the next ten years, I knew something was wrong, but not that there was anything I could do about it. So I coped the best I could. Only in the past seven years have I discovered what PMDD really is and that there are as many ways to manage it as there are women who have it, which is reported at 3-8%, and sometimes up to ten percent of all menstruating women.

PMDD is not a one-size-fits-all disorder. Even the experts can't agree on what it is, what causes it, or how to treat it. So how are ordinary women like me supposed to figure it out? But we are trying—in droves. It is for all of us that I am writing this book.

Since I started researching this disorder in earnest seven years ago, I've discovered all sorts of information that is readily available, but not all in *one* place. The number of PMDD sites that have sprung up in the past two years alone, since PMDD was included as a full-blown mental disorder in the DSM-V, or the bible of the American Psychiatric Association, is overwhelming. But what I've noticed is each site has its own slant/angle/agenda, and no one site is a resource for all things PMDD, which would allow each woman to fully research her individual options.

So I decided to create a site with that goal in mind. To have one site that connects with other legitimate sites (as opposed to, say, advertisements disguised as websites) and would allow women the opportunity to figure out for ourselves what applies in our cases and what doesn't. I know what works for me. But I also know that what works for me may well not work for millions of other women—so telling you what works for me is a shot in the dark at best.

Still, there needs to be a reliable place where we can come together to sort through our PMDD issues. Thus my blog, *Living on a Prayer, Living with PMDD* was born. I included the words Living on a Prayer, because for many years, even before I found faith and discovered the power of prayer—I felt like that was exactly what I was doing—living on a prayer.

Faith has been a vital part of my journey toward understanding myself and my PMDD. I wouldn't have been able to reach the level of wellness I have without it. That's not to say faith is the only thing that will get you through it. Just that it helps enormously, and you might want to try it. But whether you believe in a Divine Power or not, you still need faith in *something* to manage your PMDD.

I say manage because despite what countless websites and medical professionals might tell you, **there is no cure for PMDD**. The most you can hope to do is manage your symptoms, maybe send those symptoms into remission for a while. But to do that you DO need faith in something—faith in yourself.

Nobody knows what's going on inside you better than you do. Nobody knows your mind better, or your body. Don't let *anyone* tell you differently, especially medical personnel who won't take the time to work with you to achieve wellness.

You *know* when something is not right. You know when you're not being yourself. You know when you're not feeling 100%. You might not know why, or what you can do about it, but in the deepest part of your being, you *know* you have a problem—and that you need help to manage it.

My first step toward managing my PMDD was to get to know myself, to *like* myself, to trust myself, and to learn how to listen to *myself*—and not to anyone or anything outside my body. That's not to say I don't listen to the experts. I still read everything I can find on the subject. But I filter that information through my mind and heart and body based on my forty-plus years of experience with PMDD and what I now know about myself. I listen to my body when I try any new practice or treatment, and fine tune things as I go.

As of this writing I am not PMDD-free, but I am drug and

surgery free and able to function every day of the month. Some days I have to take it easier than others, for sure, but I'm no longer incapacitated by my PMDD and I no longer suffer from all the fallout that PMDD causes in our lives such as broken relationships, unhealthy addictions, and the overwhelming negativity that sabotages our joy, creativity, and positive thoughts.

In my blog, I've shared my journey with PMDD. In this book, I want to provide some tools and resources you can use to help you to have happier relationships with the people closest to you, and the ones you want to spend your time with.

I also want to make sure you know that while PMDD is not normal, you are still a normal woman with normal thoughts and emotions, needs, hopes, dreams, and desires. It is the PMDD that magnifies these normal thoughts and emotions, hopes, dreams, needs, and desires, and the responses to them (by others) and makes you overreact in irrational and extreme ways. But the root hopes and fears, worries and concerns, issues and emotions that you face each and every day are the same as those of any other woman.

It is the PMDD that is abnormal. Not you. **You are not your PMDD.** You are not damaged or broken. Quite the opposite. My hope is that by the end of this book you will believe this in your heart and will have come to accept that while PMDD is something you must deal with, *it is not who you are*.

You are so much more than your PMDD. And in the pages to come, I hope you will come to understand why.

Chapter One

———◆———

The Most Important Relationship
You Will Have

Outside of your relationship with God, but that is not the focus of this book. This book is about you, and your PMDD. So here goes:

Relationships Begin With You

Relationships are hard, no matter who you are, or what your situation is. Relationships for a woman with PMDD can be almost impossible to sustain, because, due to our hormonal fluctuations, we're literally a different woman every day. We feel differently, think differently, and act differently *every single day*.

There's an old joke that goes: A woman marries a man thinking he will change. A man marries a woman thinking she won't change.

Unfortunately, both end up being disappointed.

Change is inevitable. That's our only guarantee in life, short of death and taxes. Life comes and goes in cycles, and nothing stays the same. You will change, I will change, and your family and/or partner will change. Your circumstances, situations and environments will change, physically, mentally, emotionally, spiritually, financially, and otherwise. Accept that now, and you'll be a lot further ahead of the game than most of us.

Why? Because nobody likes change, even when it's for the better. Change takes work, motivation, and concentration, whether it's a change we embrace (like maybe a new move or a new job or a new baby), or a change we resist (like maybe a new move or a new job or a new baby). It all depends on your perspective.

But in general, we like to be comfortable in our surroundings and relationships. We like knowing what we're in for, how our day will go, what we're up against, what to expect. A certain stability gives us a good foundation for dealing with all the surprises life throws our way, be they blessings or challenges.

A woman with PMDD, just like anyone else, likes to have stability in her life. Unfortunately, that's not a luxury we can rely on, given the rocky ups and downs caused by our menstrual cycles. And what affects us, affects the people around us—in particular the people closest to us. Our friends, relatives, and significant others. It takes an incredible amount of inner strength to be the kind of woman we want to be, especially when our brains won't work right. Even the most patient and loving person loses it at times—think of Jesus in the temple, ranting at the moneychangers.

So how can you expect yourself to be any better, or different?

Take a moment right now to stop and think about that.

You don't have to be perfect. Remember that.

And you certainly don't have to be perfect to have the kind of relationships you want.

To those who have asked if it is even possible for a woman with PMDD to have a solid, steady, loving relationship, the short answer is yes. The longer answer is it will take work on both sides of the relationship. In the first half of this book, we will focus on you and what you need to do for your relationship health and wellness. In the second half, we will move on to what your partner can do to help the relationship work better.

The first step is awareness. You have to realize and accept that your PMDD is a part of you, and isn't going to go away, not without you making some serious changes in your life. The more awareness you have, the better you will feel, but the PMDD never really goes away. You have to stay vigilant, because when you slip, as we all inevitably do, there's a very good chance your symptoms will return, and sometimes worse than before.

So how do you gain this awareness? By taking the time to listen to your body and be good to yourself. Your first and most important relationship in this life needs to be the relationship you have with *yourself*. You've got to take care of you, before you can take care of anyone else. You've got to love yourself, before you can truly love someone else, no matter who that someone might be. It can be a child, a parent, a partner, a lover, a friend. If you want to have any hope of having that relationship succeed in a healthy way...you have to put you and your wellness needs first. You have to take care of you. I will have a section on self-care later on in this book, because many of us are so conditioned to take care of others first, that we haven't the foggiest idea of how to put ourselves first without feeling enormously guilty, or without making those around us feel enormously guilty.

Nobody ends up happy when that happens.

Most women with PMDD spend a lot of time hating ourselves. Beating ourselves up, for things over which we have no control—in particular the way our PMDD negatively magnifies our thoughts and moods, which then affects our words and actions. I don't need to tell you how the cycle goes. You've already been there, done that, at least once a month for as long as you've had PMDD.

So the first thing you have to do, no matter how awful you may think you are, or might have been to yourself or others in the past, is to stop beating yourself up. Just stop it. Right here. Right now. Stop it. You are who you are, and that's where you start. Don't be dragging all that baggage from past PMDD episodes along with you. Let go of it and start anew. Today is a new day, and today you are going to be good to yourself, if only for a few minutes.

Because change is hard, and works the best if you do it in baby steps. Not many of us can suddenly start shoving everyone else aside to carve out time to be good to ourselves. We have commitments and responsibilities, and if we're very lucky, people who depend on us for some measure of support, comfort, and stability.

But we also have a commitment and a responsibility to ourselves, to be as good to ourselves as we can possibly be. That doesn't mean chucking it all and hopping the next plane or cruise ship to some exotic destination, as tempting as that sounds. It just means take a few minutes, either at the beginning or the end of your day (or even in the middle, if you miraculously find yourself alone for a few minutes with nobody wanting or needing something from you) to remember what it is that makes you happy.

The choices are as limitless as the number of people reading this. Each one of us has at least one thing in this world that makes us truly happy, probably a couple dozen such things if we take the time to think about it, but for now, just start with one. What is it that makes you happy?

Write it down on a piece of paper. Studies show that goals are best achieved if written down...even if nobody ever sees them but you. Seriously. So write it down. Right here. Right now. And don't you dare feel the slightest bit foolish for doing so. We're talking about you, and you are the most important person in the room right now. There is nothing, and I mean nothing, to be nervous about or ashamed of for having hopes and dreams. Period. It's those who don't have any hopes or dreams we need to worry about, and that is not you, or you wouldn't be reading this book.

Now...what do you need to do or change in your life to make that situation/goal/achievement happen? How far are you right now from making that happen? What do you need to do *right now* to get there? Is it something you do, or something you want to do for someone else? Is it some way of being? Some habit you want to start, or stop? If it's something you do, then what do you need *right now* to do it? What is that first step? That's all I want you to worry about *right now*.

Do you need ingredients? Supplies? Or do you just need to pick up the phone and call someone? Send them a letter or card? Maybe an email. Texting is out. You don't build relationships by texting. Texting has its purposes, but building relationships is not one of them. To build solid relationships you need to at least use your voice, and if at all possible, be face to face.

That said, do you need to leave the house to go see someone? Or do you just need to cross the room?

Figure out what it is you need, then figure out a time when you can do it. If you're not doing anything right now, why not get started? Make a list if you want to. Write down the first few steps. All of them if it's a simple project. Then put your list somewhere *you* will see it often. Go to the store if you have to, to get those supplies or ingredients. If you're not feeling up to doing that, then work with what you have right around you. Do you like to doodle? Read? Pray? Listen to music? Take a bath or long, hot shower? Talk to friends? Cook? Sing? Dance? Sew? Garden? Take walks? Play tennis? Scrabble? Chess? Maybe playing with your children brings you joy. Or spending time with a pet. Spending time with your significant other, or a group of friends. Not everybody recharges best when they are alone. Some women draw energy from being around others. I am not one of them. Groups and crowds have the opposite effect on me.

The bottom line is whatever it is that makes you happy, find a way to do it. Nobody should deny you the time and space you need to soothe your spirit and settle yourself. If they try, be gentle but firm. Say, "I'm doing this for me, so that I can be a better (mother, wife, girlfriend, partner, companion, sibling, daughter, friend) to you."

Be the change you want to see in the world, and your world will change around you. But don't expect it to happen overnight. Part of the problem is we live in a world of quick fixes and instant gratification. People have come to expect things to be easy, to right themselves with the swipe of a credit card, the popping of a pill, the immediacy of a text message. With PMDD, it doesn't work that way. With PMDD, you have to work doubly hard to be the change you want to see in the world, because not only are you bumping up against the rest of the world, who most of the time is bumping back (to say the least), half the time you're fighting yourself.

But it's not really yourself you're fighting. It's your other self, or your PMDD brain. "I don't want to be like this," you say. Then don't. Stop fighting your PMDD. Stop blaming it, cursing it, and ranting about it. (Whether you're doing it in your mind, online, or in person.) Instead, accept that you have PMDD and roll with it. Start right where you are, and start being good to yourself, by honoring your body (the only one you're gonna get) and avoiding negative stimulants (like sugar, caffeine, nicotine, energy drinks, and drugs), eating right (not junk food), getting enough rest, taking the time you need to calm and settle yourself.

Get comfortable in your own skin.

Listen to your body and give it what it needs—which is not necessarily what it wants. Listen to your deepest heart of hearts, and do the same.

You know what I am talking about. You know that voice that whispers of hopes and dreams. You might have silenced it years ago, but believe me, it is still there. Connect with it, and connect with your true self again. It's the only way you are going to triumph over your PMDD self. I'm talking about doing some serious work here. Not taking a pill to mask your symptoms so you can get on with the life that makes you so unhappy to start with.

All this talk about brain chemistry and imbalances. It's probably true, but not in the way the pharmaceutical companies would have you believe. There's a whole lot more to PMDD than just a biological imbalance, and we need to stop treating it like all you need is a simple quick fix. You are a whole person, mind, body, heart, and soul. You are not simply the sum of your random parts. You are you, inside and out, and it's time you got to know you, and why you do and say and feel the things you do.

It is not easy, but it is possible. More than possible. No pills are going to put your life to rights. Only you can do that. Sure, you can do it with the aid of pharmaceuticals if you must, but the goal is to eventually stand on your own two feet.

And you can do it, because PMDD women are by far some of the strongest women I have met. We're creative, resourceful, talented, and smart. We just need to learn how to make our PMDD work *for* us, instead of against us.

That is the balance that needs to be corrected, and that correction will only come in time, and over time. A pill can't give you balance. Only you can give you that. The gift of you.

The real you, and not the PMDD you.

And as your relationship with the real you improves, little by little, your relationships with others will improve, and one day you'll realize your PMDD isn't running (or ruining) your life anymore.

~~~

So...Overcoming Your PMDD Starts With Being Good To Yourself

I am a work in progress. One thing I have that a lot of people don't have, or don't make the time for, is self-awareness. I've been digging into this PMDD shit for so long that I've finally learned how to separate my real self from my PMDD brain self. And if you think that is strange, think again. How many times have you thought of yourself as a Dr. Jekyll/Mr. Hyde character? You can separate yourself from your non-PMDD self just as easily as you separate yourself from your evil PMDD twin. All it takes—and you're going to get tired of me saying this by the end of the book—is awareness. Self-awareness, to be exact.

Self-awareness means I'm constantly checking in with myself to see how I am feeling, and trying to determine the reasons for why I am feeling the way I am—if it could possibly be my PMDD acting up (based on where I am in my cycle—Day 1 - ?) or if it's something else.

In doing this, I've learned I'm super sensitive to just about everything I eat, drink, and breathe. For instance, yesterday I went to get my hair cut. This morning I woke up with a sore throat and congested cough. Am I coming down with something? No. It's a reaction to all the chemicals I inhaled while getting my hair cut. All I have to do is drink plenty of fluids today and I will be fine.

So I'm constantly weighing, measuring, sifting, adjusting. If I feel a little off, I ask myself—what's new? What did I do differently today or yesterday? Where did I go that I don't usually go? What did I eat or drink that I don't usually eat or drink? What stresses did I encounter that I don't usually encounter?

By constantly doing this, I'm able to detect patterns, and learn what (and who) to avoid. For instance, just going to church gets my sinuses flowing. I can smell the cloud of perfume ten feet away from the front door. The same thing can happen in restaurants, theatres, sporting or music events. This doesn't mean I don't go to those things. It just means I'm aware of what can happen, and if I feel a little funky afterwards, I know why.

Of course, to be able to discern all of this, you have to be as drug free as possible. If you have a serious medical condition that requires medication to keep you alive, then you have no choice but to take it and allow it to blunt your body signals. But to treat PMDD, I am not a fan of either contraceptives or antidepressants. The main demons we deal with in PMDD are anxiety and depression. Anxiety and depression are also known side effects of the current drugs approved to treat PMDD.

Why would we choose to take a drug that creates the very same symptoms we are already experiencing? Tell me how that makes sense.

This is not the book for me to get into the subject of the

drug trials used to get antidepressants and birth control pills approved for treatment of PMDD, and the meta-analyses performed since, but I will do so in my publications *PMDD and Contraceptives*, and *PMDD and Antidepressants*. Please check my blog to see if these publications are currently available. In the meantime, read the flyer that comes with your prescriptions, or go to Drugs.com or Rxlist.com and look up your drug(s). You'll see all the potential side effects listed there.

Know what it is you are putting into your body, and how it can affect you. Then, when you're listening to your body, and feel a little off, you can better determine if there is something going on with you, or if it could be due to the drug.

I'm determined to live my life drug free. Because I feel this way, even taking two ibuprofen affects me as much as say, taking a narcotic painkiller would affect someone who isn't used to it. Oddly enough, since the birth of my son—a major hormonal event—anything I take that is supposed to make me drowsy tends to have the opposite effect. I can't take decongestants at all. Narcotics, like Tylenol with Codeine, forget it. I'll be up all night. Same deal with morphine.

I've gotten so sensitive that even certain foods affect me strangely. It sounds crazy, I know, but what's really happening is just a strong bio-chemical reaction that when processed in my brain affects my moods. These reactions can include irritability, weepiness, anxiety, lethargy, depression, and sometimes non-PMDD related bliss or even euphoria. All of these biological responses are created by hormones. All can be explained scientifically.

I believe there are many women out there just like me.

Women who haven't been blessed with the time and opportunities I have had to sit down and be still long enough to try and figure out just *What in the world is going on in my body and brain?* We live in such busy times, running from one commitment to another, taking care of our families, conditioned by our culture, society, and religious beliefs to serve others and place our own needs last.

This drastically affects our health and well-being, but since we are so busy all the time, we don't have the time (or energy) to figure out what's wrong, why we feel so out of kilter, maybe even miserable most of the time. And then our cycle kicks in, with our PMDD, and everything goes haywire. We scream, we yell, we snap, and have wild mood swings. We lash out at loved ones and coworkers and store clerks and other drivers, and then, if we haven't found a way or two to numb our conscience, we feel badly about our behavior and find ways to beat ourselves up and/or try to make amends if we can. We spend so much time trying to make it right with people, or beating ourselves up and engaging in even more destructive behavior, that we get even further run down and behind.

And then, like clockwork, the cycle begins again. So we look for quick fixes, anything that will keep us in motion, fulfilling our commitments and obligations, keep us awake and moving long enough to get everything we need to get done that day before we crash in front of the TV or into bed, exhausted, grateful another day has ended and we have somehow survived.

It's no way to live. So several years ago I made the effort to strip my life down to what's important to me, and just focus on that. One of those things was my physical health and wellness. I figured if I could just take care of that—the rest of it would take care of itself.

Little did I know how hard "just doing that" or "just taking care of my health" would be. It's no wonder more people don't take time out to do the same.

But I'm a persistent soul, and determined to figure this PMDD thing out. What I present in this book are things I've learned along the way. They might apply to you, they might not. Every woman is different, and, like I said, due to our menstrual cycles, each of us is just a little bit different every day. That makes us mysterious and exciting, not bitchy and crazy. That makes us worth taking the time to get to know.

That makes YOU worth knowing.

So take the time to get to know yourself, physically, mentally, and emotionally. Emotionally, because you have to know what emotions are being caused by your PMDD, and what emotions are normal and natural for you to be feeling. Contrary to popular belief, women are allowed to get upset, become irritated, annoyed, and angry. It doesn't always have to be PMS or PMDD causing it, and we shouldn't have to put up with snide comments about it being "that time of the month again" every time someone else behaves badly and we express our disappointment in that.

It's about accountability, and knowing yourself enough to know when it's your fault, and when it's not. I'm not interested in taking the blame for things that aren't of my own doing. Are you? I make enough mistakes, without taking on the added burden of someone else's imperfections.

For example, a few weeks ago I was feeling just plain blah.

No energy, no willpower, no motivation. I wondered if it was my PMDD come to roost for a while, but no, PMDD comes in cycles. This had to be something else. My thoughts were validated when my PMDD did arrive, and whew! It was like the difference between night and day. For just a couple of days, I sank into that abyss of despair, and knew the difference. Clearly, on those other days, there was something missing in my body that needed to be boosted…what that was I never found out, because it went away on its own, but I now know that particular lethargy is not my PMDD.

I also know my PMDD is not me. And so I've learned to set the PMDD aside when it comes. I know it's there, and it would very much like to take over my day, but I won't let it. I acknowledge that it's present, and that I'm not crazy, and I warn my loved ones that I'm having a bad day and it has nothing to do with them—but it would be best to avoid me for a day or two.

With that in place, I go about my business, and get as much done as my energy level allows. If I need to take a nap, I do it. If I need some quiet time, I take it. If I need to eat some carbs to boost my serotonin levels…I do it. Guilt-free. That's the key. Never feel guilty about taking time to care for yourself. If you were a diabetic, would you feel guilty giving yourself a shot of insulin? Would you feel guilty caring for someone else's well-being?

Then why don't you deserve as much care and comfort as they do?

So the next time your cycle comes around, give it a shot. Just take a deep breath and refuse to give in. If you lose your focus, take a deep breath and focus again. Nobody gets it right the first time. Or every time. Cut yourself some slack until you get the hang of it. Know that you are stronger than your PMDD, and it's time you let your PMDD know it.

You *can* channel your rage and anxiety and depression into strength and calm and control with simple awareness and time and practice. It won't be easy, not at first. It's a whole lot easier to just give in and go with the flow. But where has that gotten you?

Chapter Two

---◆---

Learning to Treat Yourself Well

Relationships - Learning to Treat Yourself Like a Friend

I've said it before and I'll say it again. Relationships begin with you. The most important thing for a woman with PMDD is to have a good relationship with yourself. Obviously I have a good relationship with myself, or I wouldn't be writing this book. One of the best things I've learned along the way—and you can feel free to adopt this mentality at any time—is "What you think of me is none of my business."

It's what I think of me that matters, and as long as I am happy with me, as long as I like and respect myself, that's what counts.

Surprisingly, adopting this belief didn't turn me into a self-centered egomaniac. I think that was always my greatest fear...if I put myself first, won't I turn into some kind of monster who doesn't care about anybody but me? Then everybody will *really* hate me. (Because we all know women with PMDD regularly think everybody hates us.)

I think that's why I put off putting "me" first for so long. As women, we're socialized to put everybody else first. Love means doing for others. It's how we get love, how we give and show love, how we determine our worth in the world.

Or at least that's what we're raised to believe. But the Bible says to love your neighbor as yourself. An excellent blog post on the subject can be found if you Google Why does the Bible say to love yourself? | Faith + Hope + Love. It provides eight specific quotes from the Bible that say to love your neighbor as yourself. Having read them, in *my* opinion, to love my neighbor as myself now means to love others *as much as* I love myself.

Not more, not less.

To do that, I have to love myself first.

Loving yourself is hard when you have PMDD. You do and say things you regret all the time. But think, just *think* about all that energy wasted in beating yourself up. Think about all the good and positive things you could be doing with your time and energy instead. What would happen if you just acknowledged your mistakes, did what you could to make amends, accepted that you'd done your best with the information you had at the time, and then got on with your life?

Can you imagine how different your life would be?

So the first step to loving yourself is to accept yourself as you are, right here and now. Are you in the middle of a bad episode, or are you doing well today? Is your day just so-so? That's fine, too. Start right where you are. If you're having a bad day, what can you do right now to make your day a little better? Take a nap? Call a friend? Eat some chocolate? Read a book? Watch a movie? Make a cup of tea and just sit there feeling miserable for a while?

Then go ahead and DO it.

Nobody says you have to be happy all the time. I don't know anybody who is happy all the time. And there's nothing wrong with giving yourself a little down time, a little pampering, to help you get back on your feet again.

You know I have a real dislike for taking drugs. Any kind of drug. I'm all about natural health and healing. I'm especially against the unnecessary use of pain pills and antidepressants. But a friend once explained it to me this way: When you're in constant pain, when your body has gone haywire and is sending an uninterrupted stream of "I hurt" and "I feel miserable" signals to your brain, then what is the harm in taking an occasional pill to chemically interrupt that endless loop of biochemical messages running through your body? What's wrong with giving your body a little period of pain-free space to have a chance to recover itself from that constant stream of pain messages circulating through your system?

Along those same lines, if your pain is mental, as well as physical, then what is the harm in *briefly* taking an antidepressant to stop the endless loop of negative thoughts running through your brain? Just long enough to get you back on your feet again.

Maybe six months to a year. Not for the rest of your life.

Antidepressants and pain pills were never meant to be taken long-term or indefinitely. How they evolved into what they are today has more to do with market share than human health and wellness.

So, in the case of chronic **physical** pain, taking a pain pill can give you a small break in your constant misery. Just enough time for you to catch your breath and remember what it feels like to feel good again, and marshal your resources for the next wave of pain.

In the case of **mental** pain, it's possible an antidepressant can give you a temporary break from that endless loop of negative thoughts in your head. Possible, but far from a sure thing, as antidepressants have been proven to work on a lot less people than we have been led to believe.

In the case of **emotional** pain, talking to someone (a professional or friend), or pampering yourself in some way—listening to music, stroking a pet, reading a book, taking a walk, making a cup of hot cocoa—can give you that same little space between the endless loop of emotional pain you are feeling.

For spiritual pain, read a book, watch a program, listen to a motivational CD, go to a place of worship or time spent in silent prayer or contemplation can help. Just you and your Maker. Quiet time with the spirit that lives inside you.

That's being good to yourself. Whichever of these four areas is calling out to you the loudest, start there. Baby steps. Take time out to get a handle on your pain, be it physical, mental, emotional, or spiritual. If you don't do it, nobody's going to do it for you.

Because *you* are the only person who knows what is going

on inside you. *You* are the only person who knows just how hard it is to be you.

Especially on the days when you don't feel like YOU.

For instance, yesterday I was listening to my body and being good to myself. I woke up with a tremendous pain in my neck, one that had kept me awake for most of the night, so I called my chiropractor first thing. I made my first appointment in months, and then *listened* to him when he told me to go home and take it easy, instead of throwing myself headlong back into my life. I came home and took a three-hour nap, then spent the evening reading a book. This morning, I made sure I attended my slow movement and stretching class, knowing that would help to keep my positive healing energy going.

Was there a lot I didn't get done? Yes. Do I feel 100% better? Yes. Much better than slogging through the day, trying to cross half a dozen more things off my to-do list. Because my body is in pain, I need to take care of me, or I will be miserable and no fun to be around at all.

Since I started doing this unfailingly—listening to and attending to, instead of ignoring my body—I rarely have a PMDD episode to speak of. I've had a dip or two in mood that was quickly boosted by taking a walk and/or eating some healthy whole-grain carbs, but other than that my PMDD life has been on a pretty even keel for several years now.

Loving yourself comes from taking care of yourself. From listening to yourself and attending to your own needs. The more you do this, surprisingly enough, the *less* selfish you will become. Along the way, you manage to develop empathy, and realize you're not as alone in your pain as you thought you were.

So start small. Find just one way each day to be good to yourself. You would do it for a friend or loved one who needs healing. Why not for yourself?

PMDD Flashback #1

As I said in the previous chapter, I am doing very well these days at managing my PMDD, but for the purposes of this book, to show you how I used to be, I will periodically include a story from my PMDD past. These stories come from blog posts written at the time, and often while under the influence of my PMDD.

~~~

Snapping Out with PMDD

Here's but one small example of how PMDD can affect your life and or relationships. A few weeks ago my teenage son mentioned a wildly popular movie he'd seen over the weekend, and asked if I wanted to watch it with him. I love watching movies, love spending time with my son. I was thrilled he'd thought enough of the movie (and me) to ask so even though I had already seen the movie years before and didn't particularly care for it, I said, "Sure, honey, we can watch it this weekend."

Ever since he started kindergarten, we've enjoyed Movie Night every Sunday evening as a way to settle in and prepare for the week to come. So he got the movie, and brought it home. A few days later, movie in hand, he asks, "Do you want to watch the movie now?"

And I snapped out on him and told him in no uncertain terms that I did not.

I don't recall doing it. This is not me. I mean, I've watched Winnie the Pooh and Thomas the Tank Engine and Theodore the Tugboat videos over and over and over again. I've seen most

Disney animated videos at least twice, some several times. For a couple of years, I stopped what I was doing every afternoon to watch the Power Rangers.

I have watched a LOT of shows and movies I might not have felt like watching, but did so because they were age appropriate at the time.

But apparently I changed my mind this time, and I don't even remember doing so.

A few weeks later, I innocently mentioned to my son in passing that we hadn't watched the movie yet, and he looked at me and said, "That's because you said, 'I don't see why I should have to sit through a movie I don't even like just because you want me to watch it.'"

"I did?" I asked, totally embarrassed. "When did I do that?"

"A few days after I first asked you about it and you said it would be okay."

"I'm sorry," I said. "I don't remember doing that. What did you say or do when I did that?"

He shrugged and said, "I just figured it was one of your PMDD days and left it alone."

I'm glad he knew it wasn't him that caused my snappishness, but still…

"Where's the movie now?" I asked.

"In my room," he says.

"You want to watch it?"

He did. We did. It was better than I remembered. Although I also remembered why I didn't like it as it contained some subject matter I find unpleasant. In addition to that, it had a sad ending.

"You asked me to watch a movie that would make me cry?" I teasingly accused him afterwards, still sniffling.

But he was sniffling, too. It was a good movie, a good moment, and sparked a good conversation about life and death.

And I would have missed that chance to have that conversation with him because of my PMDD.

I try not to look back, but I wonder how many other opportunities like that I missed because of something sharp I said when I didn't mean to. Worse yet, I wonder how many times I hurt someone's feelings by snapping out and don't even remember it.

Because that's part of PMDD. You get irritable, you snap at people, and *don't realize you're doing it.* You think you're behaving normally until something ugly happens, or someone who feels close enough to you or comfortable enough with you gently points out you may be having an episode. (Which nine times out of ten you will vehemently deny until you realize they are right.)

Or, before either you or they are aware that you have PMDD, they may be less gentle or understanding, and may simply shout, "What the hell is wrong with you?"

You don't know, they don't know, and the relationship starts to strain at the seams. If you don't get help, unless your friend or partner is a total saint or a doormat, the relationship falls apart.

Sound familiar?

Well, take heart in knowing it takes two to make a relationship work and it takes two to bring one to an end. It isn't and wasn't completely your fault. When you're having an episode of PMDD, certain factors are out of your control.

That's an explanation, not an excuse. (I will say this over and over and over again, so get used to it.) You still need to go back and make amends if you've hurt someone you care about while your brain was not firing properly. You don't need to beat yourself up over it. Your rage and irritability and emotional outbursts during an episode of PMDD are as uncontrollable as an allergic reaction. Doesn't make them or the consequences from them any less painful, but neither does it mean you have to drown yourself in guilt afterward. You simply apologize and do what you can to make up for it.

If your loved ones really love you, they will understand and accept that there are times when you just aren't yourself.

If you really love them, you'll do everything in your power to see that those episodes are few and far between.

Chapter Three

————◆————

Befriending Yourself

Relationships - How To Be A Friend To Yourself

Again, to love or be a friend to others you first need to love or be a friend to yourself. What exactly does that mean? I mean, if somebody told me I need to be a better friend to myself I'd probably get annoyed. What are you talking about, be a better friend to myself? I treat myself just fine, thank you. Give me some real advice, why don't you? Don't just spout platitudes like you've got it all covered.

So I started thinking about it. What does that even look like, being a friend to myself? How does one go about doing such a thing? The first answer I came up with was: Easy to say, hard to do. And why is it so hard? Because it requires thought. And most of us barely have time to think anymore. We live in a world of instant this, instant that. Technology has sped our lives up so much that half the time we don't know whether we're coming or going. All we know is we're racing here and there, trying to get everything done that we think needs doing.

But we're not really thinking, are we? We're just doing. We're doing all the things we've been conditioned to do since the cradle. We've accepted that this is how it is, this is how it has to be, and the last thing we have time for is to think about being good to ourselves. That, we leave up to the others in our circle, be it friends, family, or co-workers.

Wrong approach. Because everyone else is just as busy as you are, and people are only going to treat you with the same amount of care and respect that you give yourself. So to be good to yourself, the very first thing you have to do is SLOW DOWN. This goes against the grain, I know. If you're a list-maker, you've probably got a list that has at least 50 things on it you need to do by yesterday. You don't have time to slow down.

Instead, ask yourself one simple question: What is the best thing for me to be doing right now? *Right now* is the critical part of the question. What is the best thing for me to be doing for my health and wellness *right now*? Is it making a healthy breakfast? Reading a daily meditation? Going to the gym? Driving a parent to a doctor's appointment? Cleaning the bathroom?

That's a valid answer, because there are some of us who don't feel right or settled unless the environment around us is clean and orderly. Others don't care, so the answer would be different for them. And that's okay. But try this for a week.

Several times a day, stop and ask yourself, what is the best way to spend my time *right now*? What is the most important thing I need to take care of *right now*?

Don't just run through your days like a mouse in a maze. Take the time to become consciously aware of what you are doing, and *why* you are doing it, each and every minute—or for as many minutes as you can hold the thought, while racing from commitment to commitment, or obligation to obligation.

Maybe it's work. You need to get paid. Then be aware that you're going to work, in order to get paid, so that you can provide your family with food, shelter, clothing, or luxuries. Are you going to work for a bigger TV, a fancier cell phone, or a new stove? Are you going to work for an island vacation, a school tuition bill, or new braces? Why are you doing what you're doing, and is it the right reason and the best use of your time?

If not, then notice the gap between where you are and where you want to be, and think about what you can do to close that gap.

What about your so-called free time? Say you're at home. What is the best way you can be using your time right now? Is it changing the sheets, helping a child with homework, paying bills, or do you just need a little time out? Time out to read a book, play with the kids, call your mother, or maybe make a cup of coffee and sit down long enough to catch your breath, then jump back onto the treadmill of your life.

If you never ask yourself this question, you'll never answer it. And if you take the time to answer it, you will more than likely be surprised by the answer.

The interesting thing is once you start asking yourself this question, *What is the best thing I could be doing with my time right now?* your priorities will start to fall in line, and you'll start coming closer to where you want to be, to being the person you want to be.

I compare it to choosing a house. Many of us move into houses that are already built, and then work with what we have. But what if you had the opportunity to create your own house, to design it to have everything you ever wanted in a home? Twenty years ago, I couldn't have even envisioned the idea. I thought I had no opinions on such things.

But then I had the opportunity to design my own house from scratch, and I found out I had very definite opinions on what I wanted. It was easier than I would have thought, to go into a store and pick out tile and countertops and flooring and lights and fixtures.

But nobody had asked me before, what I liked or didn't like about my house, and so I never considered it. I just worked with or around what I had.

The same can be said of your life. What do you like or not like about it? What would you change if you could? What would you design differently if you could start from scratch? This takes us back to the very first section in this book. Start now. Start where you are. Start by taking a moment here and there to think about what you are doing right now, in this moment, and why. Then choose what you want to be doing next, and move in that direction. Eventually, you'll find out you have very distinct opinions on what you like and don't like, how you do and don't like to spend your time, who you do and don't like to be around, what you do and don't like to do or eat, what gives you energy and life—and what drains you of both.

But to do that you have to start taking the time out to ask yourself one simple question: What is the most important thing I could be doing for myself *right now*?

Is it taking a few deep breaths, is it eating an orange, is it dropping a casserole off for a sick friend, or running an errand for a family member? It doesn't have to be all about you. But it does have to be about what makes you feel good inside, because when you feel good inside you're being a good friend to yourself.

Right now I need to get this section of the book done. Why? Because today is my only day to work on it this week. But at the same time my cat has jumped onto my lap, looking for some love. Do I get annoyed and throw her off because I have something else to do, or do I stop what I am doing to pet her and coo at her and give her what she came looking for?

I stop. I slow down long enough to feel the softness of her fur, appreciate the way she pushes her head into my hands, and listen to the contented rumble of her purr. I smile and use both hands, cuddling and stroking her until she relaxes and settles in my lap, happy to be with me. She knew what she wanted, what she needed, and she came looking for it. It took maybe all of two minutes. She's happy, I'm happy, and we can both get on with our day. She, snoozing on my lap, and me, continuing to type.

What would have been served by shoving her away, muttering I was too busy to deal with her right now? I learn a lot from my cats. When they're hungry they eat, when they're sleepy, they sleep. They don't worry about what's coming up next. They live in the moment and are fully present to whatever is around them, be it a sunbeam on the carpet, the sound of the can opener, or somebody at the door.

We need to slow down like that. We need to be fully present in the moment. When we're folding laundry or doing dishes, that's what we need to be doing. Nothing more, and nothing less. We need to take the time to let our thoughts roam free, not use that time to make more lists in our head or angst about things already over and done with, or what we're going to be doing twenty minutes from now. In twenty minutes, we'll deal with whatever is happening then.

When we're driving, we need to be driving, and not doing anything else, especially not texting. When we're at the store, we need to be shopping, and nothing else. When we're talking to another person, we need to be doing that, and nothing else. When we're praying, we need to be praying. The same goes for having a meal, so that we can stop and think about what we are putting into our bodies. Is it something that is good for us, or not? Or are we just wolfing down fast food while we chauffeur the kids to wherever it is they have to go and talking on the phone in between bites?

Tell me. How is that being good to yourself?

PMDD Flashback #2

A Perfect Storm of PMDD

Unfortunately, I'm one of those atypical types who has my PMDD served up in three different courses, which is one reason it took me so long to get diagnosed. All the sites and information said specifically that for it to be PMDD all symptoms must abate at the onset of menses, or when your period begins.

But mine never did. Mine came in three separate stages. Which I finally learned is possible as well. God knew I'd been living it long enough—but to see it mentioned in a book? Finally, I could go to my doctor with confidence and get diagnosed.

I often compare my symptoms of PMDD to the course of a hurricane. Pre-menstrually is the building storm, the wind and the rain, with symptoms of irritability, edginess, an inexplicable, almost ravenous hunger, and cravings for salt and three specific foods—cheese, chocolate, and oranges. I have yet to figure out why, although occasionally I get glimmers of understanding and I am sure I will find the answer some day. But for now it's enough to know that that's what I crave, and when I find myself reaching for nothing but those three foods, I know a storm is about to blow in.

On my pre-period days I also get jittery, clumsy, confused, and distracted, unable to focus on any one task for any length of time. My handwriting even changes. Usually, it's comfortable, loose, flowing. When I'm having an episode of PMDD, it's spiky, jerky, and messy. At times it looks like the handwriting of a much older woman. I'm always startled to see it come out that way, but not totally surprised, because as I'm writing my hand doesn't seem to work properly—which might also account for my tendency to drop things more than usual during those periods of time.

Anyway, the unfamiliar handwriting is one clue that something is happening in my brain. My typing is also affected. I have a friend who pointed out that I don't bother to capitalize in my emails when I am having an episode of PMDD and I don't do a lot of smiley faces. It's as if to do either would take too much effort.

So in my case first comes the storm of irritability, anger, and rage. Snapping out at the drop of a hat. Lashing out at someone who didn't say anything out of the ordinary, but just struck me as wrong. Feeling under attack and wanting to hit someone, anyone. Just give me a chance. Not a reason, but a chance. I call these my wanting to "drink, smoke, and be bad" days. Impulsive behavior does its best to take over, and I can fully understand in those days why some women go out and do completely irresponsible things they later regret. I've felt like doing so more times than I can count, and have complete empathy for those who give in to these bizarre urges. If I didn't have a core of faith inside me that keeps me anchored in good times and bad, I would go out and do the same.

Usually the worst thing I ever did was go shopping and buy all sorts of things I didn't need or never wore. If I were to look at my credit card statements for those time periods I'm sure I would see a pattern of spending that coincides with the premenstrual portion of my PMDD episodes. Fortunately, now I understand what is happening and stay home on those days instead of going shopping. Because inevitably the bill would come, and I would wonder why on earth I had done such a thing.

When I worked as an analyst for the government, on my pre-menstrual days I would suddenly notice that I hadn't received a response on this project or the other, and would call up the parties in question and remind them I was waiting to hear from them. On any other day it wouldn't have bothered me. People get busy, people go on vacation, people have priorities, people forget. In the overall scheme of things, my projects were never that vital. Most of the time, I was tolerant and flexible.

But on a PMDD day, everyone I came across was either incompetent or personally holding me back from untold success. I might not rant at them directly—after all, even on my worst days I knew you catch more flies with honey than vinegar—but I would complain to anyone else who would listen about how I seemed to be the only person around who could get things done and do them right. I had no tolerance for the slightest delay or mistake.

Then my period would come and I'd be miserable in a new way for a couple of days. Cramps, backaches, and pain that sometimes radiated as far down as my knees, and made me feel like I wanted to throw up. Breathing hurt. I would lie very still, hot pack pressed to my lower abdomen, which felt like someone was slowly trying to pull my insides out with a three pronged gardening tool. Every. Single. Month.

That, if you want to believe it, was the eye of the hurricane. The first two days of my period.

Then the sadness kicked in. On Day Three. Always on Day Three. If it was going to come, that would be the day. It didn't always come, still doesn't. Now I know it has to do with whether I release an egg or not that month. No egg, no sadness. Woo hoo! Party time.

Not quite. But at least it's a lot more pleasant around here when the sadness doesn't come. Because when it does, I'm tired all the time, my head feels like it has an iron band around it, and I sigh incessantly—big, deep sighs like the weight of the world is on my shoulders—because for me, it is. Most everything looks hopeless, every good idea I had during the month goes to shit, I want to weep at every turn, you don't dare tell me a joke or tease me, and I spend a lot of time wondering why I even bother.

During this phase of my PMDD, I used to beat myself up incessantly over the people I had snapped out at the week before. Now, at least, I don't do that anymore. I know I didn't mean it, and in most cases it doesn't get that far anymore, because I have a much deeper awareness of what is going on and can catch myself in counterproductive behavior.

Now, when I catch myself starting to snap out, I apologize and explain I am having a bad day. Most of my friends know what that means. If the person isn't my friend, it's okay to leave it at an apology without an explanation. By all means, if at all possible, never ruin a perfectly good apology with an explanation. You don't need to justify yourself or your behavior. You only need to acknowledge it, apologize for it if the incident warrants an apology, and move on.

But back then, as I said, I would beat myself up incessantly. This only intensified my sadness and made me feel like a totally worthless human being. My friends couldn't possibly be my friends. They wouldn't be my friends if they knew the real me. How would I ever find anybody to love me if I was so impossible to be around? Yada yada yada. You know how it goes.

The bottom line is the first part of my personal hurricane is the moody, bitchy, out of control part. Then would come the eye of the storm and two days of solid pain but surprisingly clear thinking. Fortunately, now, as I begin to enter menopause, it's just the clear thinking part, and a huge surge of positive energy. It's a definite reprieve in the storm.

Then the sadness comes. Dysphoria. The first D in PMDD. My depression. Or The Fog, as I call it. Back then it was devastating. How could anybody not hate me? Now I am able to separate myself from it and while it is still not pleasant, I know I am not my depression. I rest, relax, take it easy, spend time reading or listening to music or doing something quiet and non-demanding, secure in the knowledge that my PMDD will pass. I do what I can to help it pass sooner. I take walks, take naps, eat right and take supplements. I do not allow my negative thoughts to take over. In fact, I smile at them, knowing I know better. God does love me and so do the people in my life. My ideas are good ones and I am full of creativity. I am strong, capable, and competent. I'm just running a little slower than usual today. Just a tad off my stride. It will pass and I will be fine.

And I am. One day The Fog lifts, and it's back to the hectic pace of my life as usual—until the next wave of cravings and irritability hits.

Chapter Four

Comments from Readers

A Perfect Storm of PMDD is one of my most popular blog posts. Occasionally, readers leave comments. The following are snippets of comments made after I wrote this post. I thought I'd share a random few here so you get a chance to hear from somebody besides me. Any responses to the reader from me are in italics.

᠅

With everything I've been going through these past few years and it getting worse and worse since the birth of my second son almost 4 years ago, I've been searching and searching for an explanation. I thought I'd found it in PMDD until I read that symptoms go away once your period starts. Not my case, just like you. I also start with anger and irritability and intolerance to noise and then things calm down once my period starts, but I'm exhausted. Then, 3 or 4 days after it begins, I get one day period-free then the next day, it starts up again with first-day cramps and back pain. Sadness and depression are present throughout at varying intensity. So basically, I'm myself for about a week and a half, two weeks out of every month. The rest of the time I'm this sort of monster, feeling worthless and useless, feeling like I'm a bad mother and an awful girlfriend.

~ ⁝ ~

Thank you so much for giving me hope, 30 years of the same kind of PMDD as you describe. Am also drug free for ten years after being used as a human guinea pig by so-called professionals. Being told there is no such thing as PMDD, at the same time giving me coils that release hormones, hormone replacement therapy and SSRI's at the same time.

~ ⁝ ~

I have no close friends; most people think I am crazy and when I try to explain to them I sound even crazier. So I live in isolation mostly and have to pretend I am okay when I see people. My mother has tried to have me admitted a few times. Only my son and daughter get the real me and my PMDD and if it was not for them I am sure I would have taken my own life by now. Thank you so much, you make me feel like holding on and living.

~ ⁝ ~

My heart goes out to all of you going through PMDD. You are not alone. Mine got to a point where it was affecting all my body systems. For a week and a half my

body did shut down and all I could do was sleep. I even ended up in the emergency room with a twisted bowel and I suspect it had to do with PMDD because the doctors failed to figure out why my bowel twisted. Imagine, during PMDD, I actually forget how to spell words, my cognitive skills dropped to zero ... I burst into tears when I read everyone's story because I know what PMDD can do.

~⁖~

I love the name Livingonaprayer. If it weren't for that I don't know where I'd be. I also find that my PMDD continues through my period. No major pain except for extreme achiness in my joints, almost as if my bones hurt in my legs. I also find that on around day two or three I have heightened sensitivity to sound, smell, and touch. The next day is usually a total crash. I am so tired I can barely function.

~⁖~

I know the feeling of the storm—the mental confusion and the lack of patience. I could snap at anybody for the slightest thing which is very odd because I am usually extremely passive. But I have thought the same thing, "God help anyone who messes with me at this time." It's kinda scary to think I could do something I would later regret but as the site says—we are living on a prayer.

~⁖~

I don't know if I am the only man reading these blogs, but my girlfriend's PMDD has been quite a rollercoaster ride in our

39

relationship of 3 1/2 yrs. Obviously it must be awful for her, but it certainly has put a huge strain on our relationship. She is very intelligent, beautiful, etc, and within 9 months of meeting I had proposed, just after she moved in with me. The monthly PMDD became so bad with talking about weddings etc that I eventually said I thought we should delay the wedding. Well, that created so many more problems. I didn't want to let her down, but her behavior took me by surprise every month, and I was left astounded at what had just happened.

~҂~

I am at the beginning of my journey to understand my PMDD. About 2, 3 years ago I started noticing my unexplainable bouts of depression had a pattern. Unfortunately I had no one around who had ever heard of PMDD but a couple of months ago my ob/gyn diagnosed me with PMDD and it's helped a lot. I'm in between testing Prozac and 5-HTP separately on myself to see if one will help as they cannot be taken together.

~҂~

My wife has PMDD 2 weeks each month. I can now track it on a calendar. The meanness, sharp tongue, irritability, over sensitivity to the slightest comment...it's all there each month, like clockwork. I used to make the mistake of reacting to her negativity, which results in a showdown at the OK Corral with talks of divorce, etc. etc. Now, I just keep my mouth shut, offer my help, not reacting to the negativity. It's not easy at all. My only escape is to go to the gym when it seems everything I do is wrong in her eyes. But I bear it each month because I love my wife and I know it's not her. I say she becomes Mr. Hyde once a month for 2 weeks, and I just learn to keep my mouth shut. A big exercise in tolerance and patience. If you love your wife or special someone, tolerance and patience are vital. If you don't have them, you will suffer.

~\'~

I may also suffer from anxiety separate from PMDD and sometimes I cannot escape those terrifying feelings of no control ... I'm so afraid of those who think its PMS because my only defense is "No, it's different, far more intense." "Yeah, that's what each woman says about their period." "No, really, I consider suicide once a month like clockwork, and that's not normal." "Oh, more drama..." These are conversations I've had and fear I'll have again.

~\'~

PMS is primarily physical symptoms with a little moodiness thrown in. PMDD is something else entirely. You can't be responsible for what other people think, but given the responses you presented in your comment, my guess is they simply don't care enough to "listen" to you. The fault does not lie with you. You are attempting to communicate your condition and your needs. They are not listening.

~\'~

My girlfriend would storm out over the smallest of things, and I wouldn't see her for a week. It would then take us another week to make up, by which time her next cycle would start. I ended up losing 2 well paid jobs because of all of the problems we had. We are still together, but live separately, and are trying to work things

out. **I know how hard it is for her, and she is my main concern, but it has also really affected me. I think our only long term solution is for her to have children, and then have a hysterectomy. Identical story to her mother.**

~\!/~

Is there any way to get this corrected, I am on the pill but it does not help; around that time I get psycho crazy and my husband and my fighting gets bad. I do not want my kids going through a broken home because of this. I am so torn up and do not know what to do.

~\!/~

Footnote:

The Strange Case of Dr. Jekyll and Mr. Hyde is a novella written in 1886 by Robert Louis Stevenson. According to Wikipedia, the work is commonly associated with the mental condition often called "split personality," referred to in psychiatry as Dissociative Identity Disorder, where within the same body there exists more than one distinct personality. In this case, there are two personalities in Dr. Jekyll, one apparently good and the other evil; with completely opposite levels of morality. The novella has since become a part of the language, with the phrase "Dr. Jekyll and Mr. Hyde" referring to a person who is vastly different in moral character from one situation to the next.

Chapter Five

———◆———

Relationships with Friends

Next, I'm going to talk about relationships with friends. I know everybody wants to skip to the part about Relationships with Significant Others, but really, any relationship you have with a partner, fiancé, spouse, significant other, should be rooted in friendship for the best chance to succeed. If you're already in a relationship, that's okay, you might still want to read this section if the foundation of that relationship is crumbling and you need to start building it back up again.

≈

Choosing Your Friends Wisely - Whether You Have PMDD Or Not

Okay, so we've learned that relationships begin with you, you need to be a friend to yourself before you can be a friend to anyone else, and being a friend to yourself starts with slowing down and listening to yourself, mind, body, heart, and soul.

So let's talk about friendships. Those of us with PMDD have at one time or another isolated ourselves, because we don't feel friends or family will "understand" when we are having an episode, so it's easier just to go into isolation and deal with it alone.

Easier, but is it healthier? Wouldn't it be nice to know you're still loved and people still want to be around you, even when you feel the most unlovable?

You do this by choosing your friends wisely. You do this by choosing friends who are patient, kind, compassionate, and understanding. You do this by moving away from people who are not. As a woman with PMDD, you need to look out for yourself, because—and here it comes again—nobody is going to do it for you. If this means ending or scaling back a few friendships and/or relationships, then so be it.

You have to do what is right for you. Why would you want to remain in a friendship that isn't healthy for you?

You decide who you want to have in your life, and who you don't. You don't have to cut former friends out completely. You can simply put some distance between you—see them less often, speak/email/text them less often, or speak only when you run into each other during school, church, or social events….

Just don't do anything one-on-one anymore. Especially not with someone who has ever shown you annoyance or impatience or indicated they think less of you when you have had to cancel an outing due to your PMDD. Or worse, someone who minimizes your effort to attend an event *despite* your PMDD.

Instead, surround yourself with the kind of person you would like to be. To me, that's kind, caring, giving, compassionate, and loving. I've moved away from anyone who doesn't embody the kind of qualities I want to see more of in my life. I've moved away from those who are negative, demeaning, demanding, needy, and live lives full of drama they create themselves.

Some people need a lot of drama in their lives to be happy. I'm not one of them.

I'm not saying you can only be friends with people who are the same as you...or people without any problems (is there such a person??)...not at all. I have many different friends, with all sorts of different lifestyles, problems, interests, and beliefs—but they all hold the same caring qualities in common. They have patience and understanding, tolerance and compassion, and accept when I tell them I'm having an episode and can't really participate in whatever is going on.

They allow me to talk about my PMDD openly, and even though they don't understand it, and cannot imagine what I am going through, they accept that I am going through something that is extremely painful, upsetting, and draining for me.

They don't try to:
>Talk me out of it
>Tell me to get over it
>Tell me I'm being a witch or boring or no fun to be around
>Blame me for ruining their plans

Nor do they tell me to "smile," "relax," "shape up," or

"stop being so sensitive."

And nobody, but nobody, tells me to "just think happy thoughts."

No, my friends let me be quiet when I need to be quiet, and understand if I say things that don't quite make sense.

On my part, I feel it's up to me not to snap at or lash out at my friends, and so I take full responsibility for that. If I slip, I apologize immediately, and explain that I am having a PMDD day.

PMDD is an explanation, but never an excuse.

In this way I have, over time, created a circle of friends who might not fully understand what PMDD is about, but respect and understand that *I know* what's going on, and if I say I'm having a bad day, then they accept that I am having a bad day, and don't expect or ask for more than I am able to give.

Sometimes I don't feel like going out or meeting anyone at all. Sometimes I will go to whatever it is, a meeting, dinner, lecture, concert, lunch or church, and just sit there and be quiet. Sometimes I will openly talk about what I am feeling inside, and how it completely goes against the reality of my life. I might even talk about how my negative inner thoughts reflect the opposite of what is going on in my outer life, and how that doesn't make any sense at all.

My life is very good. I have been abundantly blessed in ways tangible and intangible. I have a fully supportive family, caring and understanding friends, a warm and comfortable home, work that fulfills me, and a son who has been well-trained to deal with a woman's hormonal moods—while at the same time accepting no disrespect from me or any other woman because of those moods.

I didn't always have these things. I've been working at it for over fifteen years, slowly pruning away what (and who) no longer needs to be a part of my life, and moving into the forefront of my life what needs to stay for me to live the kind of life I want to live—calm, creative, fulfilling, and productive.

I lost touch with some friends along the way. But as I began to better understand **and accept** myself and my PMDD limitations, I gained new, more accepting and understanding friends. I also reconnected with some of my original friends in ways I never expected, while others came and went with the ebb and flow of life.

Studies show that if you hang around certain kinds of people, you will become more like them. If you surround/align yourself with hard workers, you'll work harder; if you surround yourself with positive people, you'll be more positive; if you hang with those who take an active part in maintaining their health and wellness, you'll be more active and healthier overall; if you keep company with goal-oriented people, you'll attain a few goals yourself.

In general, if you hang around successful people, you'll be more successful. At whatever you try.

The flip side of that works as well: if you surround yourself with complainers, you'll complain more; if you surround yourself with people who like to overindulge in food, drink, toxic environments or substances; you'll do more of the same. If you hang with people who do things you know are harmful to your health and wellness, *you will do more harmful things than you may personally want to*, just to fit in.

So choose the people you want to be with carefully. If you want to be well, then make friends with those who are also trying to be well. If you want to complain, then make friends with those who complain. Either way, you will have friends…

But which friends are more likely to help you make progress toward successfully managing your PMDD?

Think about it, and then adjust your life accordingly. Listen to your body, notice how you feel before, during, or after you're around certain people. Some people can get you churned up just thinking about being around them. Take time to notice who these people are in your life. Don't just go through life on autopilot, accepting whatever comes your way. That's probably what got you where you are today, and why you're reading this book.

So slow down, come to know yourself, make friends with yourself, and then choose the rest of your friends wisely. One small step at a time.

Chapter Six

———— ♦ ————

Family Relationships

Relationships - Choosing Your Family

Families are hard to deal with, any way you look at it. They consist of the people who are supposed to love you the most, care more about your welfare than anyone else, treat you more kindly than strangers, and keep you safe from the world's evils.

But they don't. In fact, they quite often do the opposite. Which leaves all of us feeling pretty damn confused. If my family is supposed to love me and nurture me, provide for my needs and keep me safe…but doesn't…then how can I expect anyone else to love and encourage me, provide for my needs, and keep me safe?

That's a question for which I have no answer. I've spent countless hours researching family dynamics, in particular during the holidays—a tense time for families in general—hoping to be able to offer some words of wisdom on the subject, and the best advice I could come up with is…**Just say no.**

That's right, just say no. If your family is toxic, then don't go to those toxic holiday events, reunions, and family affairs. Article after article said the same thing. Being the kind of person who much prefers to see everyone get along, this message disappointed me. But it trumped my research, hands down.

I have to admit, that if you follow the advice in the earlier sections of this book, about making friends with yourself first, before you make friends with others, and about choosing your friends wisely, and choosing to spend time only with those people who exhibit the qualities you would most like to develop in yourself—how many of us would choose our own families?

Some of us have families that are truly supportive, encouraging us to be the best person we can possibly be. Others are pits of dysfunctional hell. If you have PMDD, due to the correlation between childhood abuse and PMDD, chances are your family falls somewhere in the second category. This means the relationship you're in right now could be unhealthy. This only adds to your problems with PMDD. Like attracts like (even if you're opposites—you are the same in your *inability* to have a healthy relationship), and if you were abused as a child, the chances are good you will end up in a relationship that is abusive in one way or another.

Which will only make your PMDD symptoms worse.

I'm jumping ahead of myself here, because my next topic will be dealing with your immediate family…but the facts cannot be denied…studies have shown there is a strong correlation between abusive relationships of any kind, physical, mental, emotional, and sexual, and PMDD.

So if you have PMDD, chances are your extended family relationships are strained, and holiday gatherings are pure hell. Taking us back to chapter one, where I said relationships begin with you, the number one best thing you can do for yourself is to learn to listen <u>to yourself,</u> to your intuition and your body, to become more aware of your feelings about *everything*, and let them guide you.

Emotions are just that, emotions, and they will pass. But feelings, true feelings, will resonate in your body. If the thought of going somewhere and spending time with people you don't like and who don't like you fills your body with dread, churns your stomach, gives you a stress headache, puts you on edge, or makes you reach for substances that dull your pain, then yes, you need to stop and think twice about why you are doing this to yourself.

Remember, if you don't look out for yourself, nobody is going to do it for you.

If you don't set the boundaries of what you will and won't accept from other people in the way of behavior, be they family or strangers, nobody is going to do it for you. People with abusive personalities don't recognize or observe boundaries— they will push and push and push you *as much as you let them*. You can either, 1) push back—which benefits no one, 2) set your boundaries and quietly but firmly enforce them—which abusers will then call abuse since you are no longer letting them have their way, 3) simply refuse to engage by not answering (unfortunately, this method has its own drawbacks), or 4) not attend any event in which you are likely to be treated with any form of disrespect.

In the end, it all comes down to you again, and how healthy you want to be. PMDD and stress are like the chicken and the egg. Nobody knows which comes first. But they do have a strong correlating relationship, and one affects the other. How you handle stress affects your PMDD and how you handle (or don't handle) your PMDD definitely causes stress.

The best thing to do then, to get a handle on your PMDD, is to remove all sources of stress from your life. This process in itself can be extremely stressful, but in the long run is much healthier for you than taking drug after drug to solve a problem that can only be masked, but not fixed, by taking drugs—no matter what the drug companies tell you.

The same advice applies to forming or perpetuating family relationships that applies to forming and maintaining friendships—you need to ask yourself: Are the people you spend your time with people who exhibit the positive qualities you would like to have more of in your life?

If not, then why are you spending time with them?

Sometimes you have to go out and create your own family. This works, too, because once you get right down to it, a family, like a home, is a place in your heart. You can create a home anywhere, and you can create the kind of family you'd like to have anywhere as well. To do that, however, you might have to first let go of the old one. Or at least limit contact with them until you are strong enough to stand up for yourself and can comfortably deal with the stress of the situation.

Until then, they're going to keep getting to you, your

PMDD will continue to worsen, and you're going to continue to dread every family event that comes up that will be attended by people you don't really like and wouldn't choose as friends.

The choice, as always, is up to you. I can hear the "But you don't understand!" comments now.

I can, and I do. Been there, done that. It wasn't easy or fun, but I came through it stronger, wiser, happier, and healthier than I have been in years.

Chapter Seven

———◆———

How to Survive Family Gatherings

Relationships - How To Survive Family Gatherings

There are a lot of us who genuinely would like to get along with our families and have our family gatherings filled with happy memories of good times shared. There are also a lot of us, who, for one reason or another, aren't willing or ready to make any sort of break with our fundamental family ties—because without family, what are we, but alone?

Nobody likes to be alone. Especially on the holidays, when according to what we see on television, everyone else is having the time of their lives.

So in this section I want to offer some positive thoughts and information on things you can do to make your family gatherings, be they over the holidays or for any family occasion, a little more pleasant.

1. **Lower your expectations.** Most people go into the holidays with Norman Rockwell expectations and end up deeply disappointed, even depressed and suicidal. Where do most of these expectations come from? The media. Starting as early as September, advertisements abound showing happy families sharing holiday joy. Keep in mind that these advertisements are designed to sell you products, and are not a realistic representation of what goes on in most families. Just like rail-thin runway models are not true representations of the average woman, warm and fuzzy advertisements with everyone laughing and smiling around a holiday table as they pass the food and drink are not true representations of a holiday family gathering. They are somebody in advertising's image of an *ideal*—and ideals are extremely hard to reproduce in everyday life.

So don't blame yourself if your holiday event falls short of the idealized version you see on TV. This is tantamount to blaming yourself for not having a body as hot as your favorite movie star's. Looking good is what they get paid to do. If you got paid to look that good, you would, too. Any woman can look sexy with the right hair, clothes, and make up. If you don't have access to the same spas, trainers, dieticians, life-coaches, personal chefs, housekeepers, nannies, drivers, and secretaries or assistants they do, then how can you expect yourself to look as good as they do?

The same goes for the happy families on TV. If you don't have access to the same funds and props and wardrobe and production crews that they do, how can your family holiday be as picture perfect as they portray theirs to be? They probably don't even know each other. They're just a bunch of strangers *acting* like a happy family.

Don't fall for the hype. Work with what you have, and stop trying to imitate some marketing specialist's unrealistic image of what *your* holiday gathering should be like. For instance, for Thanksgiving this year my husband and I tried out a new recipe for veggie chili, made cornbread, bought some ice cream, invited one (one!) friend over, and had a great time. This same friend and I used to do the whole turkey dinner thing with a big group of friends, which was fun at the time, but since then have shifted to more low key activities.

For Christmas, we went our separate ways. No harm, no foul. For Easter, my husband and I spent the weekend in a lakeside cabin with different friends, from my high school.

It's all good.

2. **Arrive with a smile and determination to look for the positive throughout the day.** If someone brings up a topic you'd rather not discuss, just smile and say, "Gee, I really haven't thought much about that lately." Then excuse yourself to head off for the food and or drink table, maybe ask if there is anything you can bring back for them. Deflect, divert, disarm. (If you're already at the table, pick up the nearest serving dish and offer some food. "Would you like some more mashed potatoes?" Switch the focus to them, in a polite, non-threatening way. Don't let them get your goat.) Once you've returned with whatever they might have asked for, just smile and say, "Here you go," and then be on your way. Either way,

the uncomfortable topic has been diverted.

3. **Use the event as an opportunity for growth as a person.** Practice the skills of patience, kindness, tolerance, acceptance, and/or self-control. Congratulate yourself every time you manage to take the high road and not snap out at the person who is trying to get you to lose your cool, either deliberately or inadvertently. Use the occasion as an opportunity to learn about how and, as I said in chapter three, who you "don't" want to be.

4. **Set your intention to have a good time, no matter what.** Do everything in your power to get a good night's sleep beforehand. Read up on prayer or positive thinking and prepare yourself to view the gathering as a "spiritual" event. One in which you know your spirit will be challenged, and you refuse to let anyone shake your good mood. One of the best books I've read that has to do with dealing with difficult people is *Thank You For Being Such a Pain,* by Mark Rosen.

5. **Eliminate three words from your vocabulary for the day -- Always, Never, and Ever.** Try it. Practice in advance. As in so many other areas, awareness is the key. Become more aware of these "conflict coals" and do your best to not add any more to the fire. Or, as an exercise in self-entertainment, start to notice how often others use these coals of conflict to fan the flames of family discontent.

6. **Stay sober.** I know this is a hard one, because a lot of people use alcohol to get through the day, thinking it's the only way they will be able to deal with it, but in truth alcohol only contributes to the problem, because it magnifies whatever issues are already on the table, or lurking just beneath the surface. Besides, a woman with PMDD needs to stay away from alcohol.

Like stress and trauma and abuse, alcohol only makes your PMDD symptoms worse. If you must drink, down a full glass of water in between each alcoholic beverage to both hydrate and pace yourself. My personal philosophy is when you get to the point where you feel like you "really want" another drink to keep that buzz going—the buzz is already on and it's time to start backing off or you're sure to regret it come morning.

7. **Don't choose sides in any conflict that develops.** Period.

8. **Stay away from discussions involving sex, politics, and religion.** Arrive prepared with alternate topics to bring up…bring (or bookmark on your phone/tablet) photos of the kids or your last vacation. Anything important to you or your family that you'd like to share. Try not to get your feelings hurt if your efforts to share are brushed off, ignored, or dismissed. Congratulate yourself for at least having the willingness to try.

9. **Invite a friend or two** who has nowhere else to go for the holiday dinner. Sometimes bringing new people into the situation will help to keep unruly relatives on their best behavior. Or will at least make them consider restraining themselves in the presence of guests.

10. **Drive separately, so you can escape if need be.** If you can't leave the house, then leave the room. Go into the kitchen and see if you can help there. Busy yourself with clearing plates and empty drink glasses/cans. Or just go and refill your own (preferably non-alcoholic) drink. Maybe spend some time in the bathroom, practicing deep breathing exercises. Go for a walk if you can. While you're in the bathroom or on that walk, text or call a friend you've arranged to contact beforehand

if things get dicey. Enlist some moral support, and do it guilt-free. If no friends are available to text, there are always PMDD groups on Facebook you can vent to. There is usually someone online 24/7.

11. It may well go against the grain, but if you feel you absolutely must go to the family gathering, then go and **aim for one positive encounter during the event, and build from there.** Next time aim for two, and privately celebrate your successes. It might take a few years to get where you want to be, but if this is your family, or your partner's family, you'll have as many years as you need to work on it.

12. Another sanity-saving option is to **arrive late and leave early.** Limit your time with your relatives so that whatever of the above you might be willing to try has a bigger chance of success.

When all else fails, disengage.

Because sometimes nothing less than to Just Say No will do. Plan an alternate holiday gathering/event and proceed with it guilt-free, telling your family you're taking a break and will see them next time around.

Of course, there are some of you who for whatever reason simply cannot place any distance between yourself and your tormentors—I mean, family.

Would I leave you in the lurch? Of course not. This section is for those who are unwilling—or literally unable—to take a break from your family. Recognizing that

You can't fix something you didn't break

and

It takes two to make a relationship, and two to break it,

There is only so much you can do.

If the person you are trying to connect with, be they parent, partner, sibling, or child, is not interested in having a positive relationship with you—because they do not have a positive relationship with themselves—there is nothing you can do but hang on and hope for the best.

Prayer can be very effective when you have reached this sort of impasse with someone in your life.

But I also want to stop here and make sure you realize that if you are having a bad relationship with someone, anyone, in your life, and you are doing your best to take responsibility for whatever shortcomings *you* may bring to the relationship, and it *still* isn't working...

Then the problem isn't you, and you have no business taking full blame for the faults in or failure of the relationship.

Many relationships are broken because the person you are in relationship with is also broken. They do not love themselves, and therefore literally cannot love you until they heal. This is not always their fault, this inability to love, but once people reach adulthood, how much love and goodness they have in their hearts and their lives is a direct result of their *choices* in life.

Yes, happiness is a choice. So are peace and harmony, anger and strife. People choose to be happy or sad, appreciative or critical, content or bitter, encouraging or derisive. It is absolutely true that when you have control over nothing else, over no other circumstances in your life, you still have control over your attitude. (Now, remember, I am talking about the other half of whatever relationship you are thinking about right now. This does not apply to *you*, the woman with PMDD, just yet. We will talk about you a little later.)

The fact that whoever you are having a relationship with chooses not to be happy, or not to work with you to better the relationship, or not to participate in the relationship at all, is *not your fault*. That is their fault. Fully, completely, and entirely. Do not take the blame for anyone's bad behavior but your own. Ever. Any time, any place, any where. If you are an adult, you are responsible for your own behavior. If you are under the age of 25, you can still get away with some stupid stuff, because your brain is literally not fully formed yet, and people in their twenties tend to do things without thinking them through.

That's part of life, that's part of growing up. But once you cross that line, and start heading into your thirties, it is time to start acting like an adult, or you will find yourself in relationship after relationship that does not work, and, if you have any sense of self-awareness at all, will leave you wondering why.

The first tenet of being a grown up is to take responsibility for your actions, good or bad. It's that simple. You hurt someone or their feelings, you apologize, and do what you can to make it right. You don't blame them for being too sensitive, clumsy, slow, scattered, discombobulated, or anything at all. Aside from the one to three percent of the population who are genuine sociopaths, we all know right from wrong. We are born knowing this right from wrong. In some of us, that knowing gets killed/suppressed/obliterated very early on, but for the rest of us, we *know*. We know when we are at the receiving end of something wrong, and we know when we are at the dishing out end of something wrong. That we choose to do whatever it is we are doing anyway, is exactly that...a choice. And adults take responsibility for their choices, be they right or wrong.

So if you have someone in your life who doesn't understand your PMDD, it's because they are choosing not to understand. Instead they are choosing to believe you are crazy or lazy or out of control because it suits some purpose that works for *them*, not you. (This is assuming you are making every effort to enlighten them.) They may or may not be aware of this on a conscious level, but either way, this is what is happening. If they can keep the focus on you and your failings, there is no need to look at their own. If they can get you to take the blame for whatever is wrong in the relationship, they don't need to carry their own half of the load.

Being in a relationship takes work under the best of circumstances. If you are in a relationship with someone who thinks "love is all hearts and flowers" or "relationships just happen" then you have your work cut out for you. First of all, you'll be doing double the work while they do none of it. And when something goes wrong, since you are doing all the work, you will most likely get all the blame.

Tell me how that is fair. Tell me it hasn't happened to you.

Whether it's with a friend, relative, spouse, or a child, to make a relationship work you have to spend quality time together, and you *each* must make the effort to understand the other, and to find ways to create memories that make you both smile—instead of cry. No one can tell you what, where, or how this balance in your relationship should be. This is between the two of you and no one else. You and the other party are the only ones in the relationship, and you and the other party are the only ones who can figure it out, based on your individual levels of maturity, needs, personalities, time availability, emotional awareness, you name it.

Just like every woman is different, every relationship is different. You can look across a room and see a couple you think has it all, but you don't know what goes on in that relationship. I don't care what you think you know. You only know what you see and what you are told, and even then the information is skewed unless you are told by both parties in the presence of each other. When this happens, you *still* may not get the full picture. Couples regularly leave private details out of stories they tell about themselves.

But I digress. The bottom line is the people in your life are always responsible for their own actions and choices, even when they refuse to take responsibility for them. Not taking responsibility does not mean you are no longer responsible. The responsibility is still yours, whether you accept it or not.

None of this, of course, applies to a woman with PMDD when she is in the PMDD zone. Right now we are talking about partners/relatives who are in full control of their faculties at any given moment. Once a PMDD-ing woman enters her personal PMDD zone, all bets are off until her period comes and she returns to her regular state of mind.

But guess what? Once you have a handle on your own behavior, they can't use it against you any more.

That said, no one who does not have PMDD themselves has the right to judge, blame, dismiss, discount, provoke, or otherwise torment you into making your PMDD worse. Neither do they have any right to excuse themselves for their behavior during an episode, especially while casting all the blame on you and your condition/disorder/disease/illness. Doing either—tormenting you and/or blaming you for your own torment—is abuse. Whether it's fostered by ignorance or done deliberately, it's still abuse, plain and simple.

It's so easy to blame your own failings on someone who has legitimate burdens to carry. Do not fall prey to this tactic, this emotional abuse. As women we are often socialized to accept either responsibility or the blame for the bad behavior of those around us. This is doubly true for women with PMDD. Having PMDD makes us easy targets for blame.

Do not accept that blame unless it is truly yours. Daily I hear from women about something that happened during their latest PMDD episode, and without fail, they take the entire blame for the incident, even when the other party was a total jerk.

This has to stop.

Own up to what is yours, whether you are in the PMDD zone or not. And do not for one moment take responsibility for something that did not come out of YOU.

If awareness is the first step, and it is, shedding guilt and blame is the second. The book, *Guilt is the Teacher, Love is the Lesson*, by Dr. Joan Borysenko is an excellent resource for helping you to do just that. It changed my life, and if you want to change yours, it's a great place to start.

Bonus Section:
More Tips to Survive Family Gatherings; Specifically Christmas Gatherings

PMDD and Holiday Stress

Offhand, I can think of four good sources of holiday stress: family, food, finances, and expectations. Each causes its own manner of stress, but like a toxic family with a volatile history, they all intertwine. For example: Your family has expectations that involve your finances, either via hosting a food-laden event, traveling to a food-laden event, or exchanging gifts.

Funny, but our current culture would have us believe that the more we spend, the more we care.

Is that messed up or what? Then, of course, there are the guilt purchases. You know, the sometimes extravagant but almost always expensive gifts you buy to convince someone how much you care when you won't be showing up in person. Or maybe you will be there, but you'll have to leave early, or it's the only time you've seen this person since whenever, and you feel guilty about that. Then there's the keeping-up-with-everyone-else spending. Your gift can't possibly come in at a dollar value less than the gifts "the others" are giving, or you'll look bad. So you either buy something you can't afford, or pony up your share of a gift you didn't choose and can't afford.

Above are only a few examples of generic holiday stressors. A woman with PMDD doesn't handle stress well to start with, and so when the holiday madness begins...

You can understand why all she wants is for it to be over, or at the very least, to get through it without a meltdown.

So let's stop for a minute, just stop and think. What are all these holiday gatherings supposed to be about? Connecting, making memories to hold you through until you see each other again, right? (Or, if you're all local, celebrating another year of life's ups and downs together.)

But somewhere along the way, everything shifted. Away from Jesus and family, peace and goodwill, and toward fueling a selling season that accounts for 40% of the year's retail revenue.

Connecting more deeply with friends and family is not about two months plus of frenzied shopping to see who comes up with the biggest, best, shiniest gift. It's about coming to the table well-rested and healthy, comfortable and caring. It's about making eye contact (put those electronics away!!), feeling genuinely happy to see each other, and connecting in a special way...but not in a deep, soul-sharing, forever-bonding kind of way. If you come to the party expecting that, you've fallen into the trap of unrealistic expectations, and you'll only be disappointed.

Holiday gatherings are for having lighthearted fun and making good, positive memories. If a heart to heart connection happens, consider it a bonus. But don't go into the event expecting anything more than a good time.

Happy holiday gatherings are about spending time with people who share common interests, values, and beliefs. And if that doesn't happen—which is most of the time—it's about managing to enjoy the day and company as best as you can. In a worst case scenario, it's about keeping the peace (and your peace) for as long as you and these spiritual, mental, and emotional strangers spend time together.

Not everyone is blessed enough to have a group to gather with. If you are, but can't stand to be around them, and absolutely, positively cannot escape attending the festivities, the prevailing advice is to limit your visits to a couple of hours at a time. If you've traveled long distance, take breaks to visit friends in the area, or maybe revisit familiar local haunts, or show your partner or kids where you grew up. If you don't want to do that, or don't know anyone else in town, maybe you can visit some sort of tourist attraction in the area for a break between bouts with relatives. You can offer to be the gofer who runs errands. Somebody always needs something they forgot to bring at these things. Offer to fetch it, and use the time to regroup. If you're not from the area, just take a walk or a drive to explore the surroundings and clear your head.

What is it with people acting as if there's something wrong with wanting to spend more than a few minutes alone? Could they envy your independent spirit? Wish they could break away from the herd as well? Think about it.

If you have no relatives nearby, find some friends and start your own traditions. Traditions are important, but creating new traditions can be equally important. Families no longer look the same as they did in the past. We've got single moms and dads, same sex moms and dads, bi- or multi-racial couples and children, adopted children, foster children, blended families, events where all parties and their current significant other show up, presumably for the sake of the kids—so why should family events always be the same?

Consider incorporating something new into the mix.

Maybe you can all go to church together, or to a restaurant for dinner, or to a movie or bowling after your meal. Mix up the traditional menu and try adding something new. Maybe even ditch the whole thing and have a theme party.

Or maybe you can agree to go to the big family shindig only every other year, or only participate on alternate holidays. Spend one any way you want to, (whether it be by staying home or planning a ski chalet weekend) and the next by attending a family gathering. Or schedule the family event at a different time than the official holiday. Think of all the stress you'll avoid, not scrambling out there with all the other holiday travelers.

But don't go at all if you know the event will only bring more pain and destruction to yourself and the family. Family gathering time is not the time to resolve family issues, conflicts, or make major family decisions. The discussion about your cousin's financial woes or addiction or divorce or whether or how to move someone into assisted living is NOT one you want to have at a holiday gathering. Ditto details about selling, renting, or discarding family property. True, it may be the only time you are all together, but the holiday celebration itself is NOT the forum for such undertakings. Those require a separate family meeting.

Just as the holidays are stressful for all of us, most of these suggestions could apply to anyone. To specifically address your PMDD, I'd have to return to the line of "coming to the table well-rested and healthy, comfortable and caring." If you are feeling none of these things on the date of the event, then *you are not wrong in wanting to cancel*, and if you do, please do not feel guilty or accept any blame for doing so. Would you stay home if you had the flu? Negative moods are just as contagious and can ruin a party just as easily.

Feeling guilt and accepting blame only escalate your PMDD symptoms. By staying away from the event, you are protecting the event and taking care of yourself. Nothing in this world is more important than seeing to your own health and wellness. Especially when it comes to your mental health.

What To Do if You Are the Hostess...

The short answer is: **Plan Ahead**

The longer version gets much more complicated. Because, whether you know it or not, your number one priority in this, as in all events in your life, is you and your health. So right from the outset you need to treat holiday stress like the serious risk to your well-being that it is. Some women love pulling off complicated social events at the last minute, thrive on the thrill and challenge of pulling it all together before a deadline. Women with PMDD cannot afford to be like that.

Even if you are a perfectionistic extrovert in real life and love being the hostess with the mostess—as a woman with PMDD, and for as long as you have your PMDD—you will need to rethink your strategy.

Perfectionism, deadlines, complications and surprises cause stress. If you're going to be willing to take that on, then you've got to be willing to put yourself right up there at the top of your priority list.

Yep. You. It all comes back to You. First, you have to ask yourself, **Do I really want to do this?** If the answer is yes, then proceed to the next page. But if the answer is **No,** then **Why are you even considering doing something like this?** If the answer comes down to expectations, then you have to ask yourself *whose* expectations, and what those people and *their* expectations are doing to contribute to this event. If they are *your* expectations, and yours alone, you might want to spend some time alone thinking about where those expectations came from in your past and how important they really are at this time in your life when you struggle with PMDD.

If the expectations come from someone else, then that someone else needs to step up and pitch in to help bring this event full of holiday expectations about.

Never, ever, put yourself through the motions of hosting a holiday event if your full heart and soul are not in it to start with. How does doing that benefit any of you?

So: Assuming you DO want to host a holiday event, then number one, you have to check your calendar, and if at all possible, schedule it when it is most convenient for you, and your cycle.

Next, if you regularly work out, then you must not give up one minute of that workout "me" time to do event preparation. Forget it. You must come first. You must be true to yourself and your needs during this time of added holiday stress. Doing so will keep you healthier, and when you are healthier, you will be happier, and so will the people around you.

Which is what the holiday season is all about, right? Joy, and happiness?

So daily exercise, especially when paired with something like meditation, yoga, stretching, or walking, will give you a lot less sick days, in particular less *respiratory related* sick days (as in colds and flu, bronchitis and pneumonia), than if you don't exercise.

You want to be able to enjoy your own party, right?

Exercise will also help you to sleep well, another absolute must for dealing with PMDD. And, of course, as always, watching your sugar, caffeine, and alcohol intake will help in this department. Unfortunately, any kind of buzz can seriously disrupt a good night's sleep, so you have to ask yourself is it worth it? And just six teaspoons of sugar can suppress your immune system by 50% for up to five hours. So as fun as those Christmas cookies are to make and decorate, baked goods do not do your PMDD body any favors, but especially when your stress levels are elevated already. And whose aren't the last two months of the year?

Now, assuming it is an all-day or longer affair, in addition to serving up a kick ass menu—with lots of help in making it— you'll want to have on hand several diversions to keep your guests busy. Don't rely on the boob tube alone to keep them entertained. Biggest mistake you can make.

Family time is, was, and always will be—game time. If you have a game room, orchestrate some family tournaments. Cards, pool, ping pong, whatever. People will moan and groan, but secretly they will love the competitive aspect of it. If you live in a warm climate, outdoor activities would be fantastic. Otherwise, be prepared with board games for large groups, such as Trivial Pursuit or Pictionary or Apples to Apples, or even charades. A family sing along might sound dorky, but you'd be surprised at how many will jump in, and will remember the singing times fondly.

Music is an automatic mood booster. And if you don't teach your kids the Christmas carols you grew up with, who will?

Maybe you could provide a room where you feature holiday film classics.

Another great idea is to organize an activity for charity. Have each guest bring a new item of clothing, (say, all shirts, or socks, or underwear), or various canned goods. The homeless need food and clothing year round, not just at Christmas. Together you can prepare a food basket for your local food pantry. Maybe even send out a group to deliver it to a local church or homeless shelter or refugee family. Give the kids a lesson in charitable giving.

Last but not least, if you are the one presiding over the holiday madness, then do your best to provide the tools with which your guests can have a good time, be it food, drink, games, entertainment, or other activities (maybe even crafts and baking), and then *let it all go...*

Yes. Let it all go.

Because you are not responsible for anyone else's good or bad time, attitudes, feelings, or behavior, no matter how hard they may try to convince you otherwise. *And they are not responsible for yours.*

This goes for whether you are the hostess or not, and shouldn't need to be said, because no matter what the time of year, we are all accountable for our own behavior whether we agree with that or not.

So make your choices and stand by them. If you choose to open your heart and home to others, you need to be able to do it *your* way. You need to be able to do what is right for you, and what feels right in your heart.

Actually, I think once you start to do this, your holidays will automatically become less stressful.

And that would be a wondrous gift for all.

Chapter Eight

———•———

General Wrap-up on Relationships
(before we start getting specific)

It's Not Personal, It's Just Your PMDD

Okay, we've covered your relationship with you, learning to treat yourself as well as you would a friend, how exactly to have a relationship with yourself, choosing your friends wisely, avoiding relatives who are toxic to you, and tips to get along with them if you do choose to attend or host family functions.

Now we're going to look at your relationship with another aspect of your family—the people you live with every day.

This could be any combination of people and or ages. Mother/guardian and children; parents and/or siblings (you, living with your parents and siblings); adult woman living with parents; adult woman caring for parents; roommates; mother, partner, and children and/or stepchildren; childless couples; same sex couples, you name it. But these are the people we are closest to physically, if not emotionally. It would be nice if we were as emotionally close to them as we are physically, but for any number of reasons that often isn't the case.

Stress at home is bad enough, but for a woman with PMDD, it can be the key element that prevents you from getting well, as any kind of trouble at home only exacerbates your PMDD symptoms. During a PMDD episode, we are biologically sensitive creatures, and can be sensitive to light, sound, touch, taste, and smells. This has been clinically proven. A PMDD-ing woman's five senses can be enhanced during an episode, enhanced to the point of physical discomfort and beyond, which makes us react in ways not welcome or understood by those who do not suffer such on again, off again changes in sensitivity to our senses.

Please understand this: It's biological, this shift/change that happens in our bodies, but we react to it/manifest it emotionally.

Anger has been a basic form of self defense since the cave dwellers. Our bodies are hardwired to react with some form of flight or fight (including anger and aggression) when we feel threatened.

You're having a PMDD episode and the kids are being too loud? You snap and snarl to get them to quiet down. Your head is pounding with a PMDD migraine, so you tell your beloved to shut up and turn out the lights. Both of these reactions are nothing more than self-preservation instincts kicking in. Too many flashing lights? Too much electronic noise? Same deal. Significant other giving you a hard time? Feeling like everybody wants a piece of you at the same time?

Your biological responses kick in, and you lash out in self defense.

The target of your attack responds with "What's wrong with you? I was just..."

They wonder if you're crazy. You wonder if you're crazy. Some are so mean-spirited as to taunt you and make you snap out again and again and again...

Why? Because when you're out of control, the focus is off of them. Remember that.

The best way to fight this form of abuse—and that is what it is—is to read chapter two and become your own best friend. You need to get to know yourself better than anyone else knows you, sort through what is your fault and what is not, accept your part of the blame, then change your behavior as necessary.

An example of this might be to catch yourself before you explode into anger or tears.

Or learn how to apologize when you don't.

Never apologize for "being the way I am." You are who you are. God loves you just the way you are. If your family or partner doesn't...you need to think about that.

But the very first thing you need to do is to focus on you, and get a handle on your PMDD.

For instance, if you don't catch yourself in time, and you snap out on them, apologize immediately for the hurt you caused the other person/parties. Never apologize for being upset in the first place, though. You have as much right to be upset about things as anyone else. If something is not going right in your life and it upsets you, those are valid feelings. It's how you *express* those feelings that bring your PMDD into play.

Because PMDD is biological in nature, and deals with, among other things, your stress responses. The only thing you can do to break the cycle (short of taking drugs) is to get to know yourself as well as you possibly can, and learn ways to head off any "natural as an allergic reaction" responses to stress.

If you chart your symptoms, which is a must for a woman with PMDD, you can tell when things are going to start getting dicey in your life. You can plan around those days, and plan to take it easy on those days if at all possible. Read a book, go to a movie, take a bubble bath or nap, or both. Learn to pamper yourself a little. You can also warn those you live with that those days are coming.

My house is a haven. It's where I go to find peace, to recharge, to rest and relax. It wasn't always that way, and I had to make some difficult choices and changes to get to where I am today. One baby step at a time.

But now, if I am having a bad day, all I have to do is say so, and everyone knows it has nothing to do with them and everything to do with me and my PMDD. The best course of action is to avoid me, make no demands, agree with me if I start something, and not take anything I say or do personally.

My job is to 1) stay aware of what I am doing, 2) go about my business quietly, 3) gently remind people who ask for something I can't give at that moment that I am having a bad day, 4) do my best not to start anything, and 5) not take anything personally.

The best advice for *everyone* involved is to not take anything personally.

This is not a license for you to freely do and say what you want to during an episode, but an agreement that if things should go awry or get out of hand—it's not personal. It's just your PMDD.

And if, during an episode of PMDD, others in your life behave badly, what is their explanation for it?

Think about it.

You'll soon realize it's not just you.

So stop taking the blame for everything that goes wrong in your relationships. Recognize that it takes two to have a relationship and both parties have to want the relationship equally for it to work.

I'm talking about adults here.

When it comes to kids, it should be easier to simply explain to them that Mommy is having a bad day and needs some quiet time, and it would be a really big help if they could find something quiet to do while Mommy rests so she can feel better sooner.

If your kids don't understand or refuse to honor this simple request, then a parenting class might be in order. If your partner doesn't understand or refuses to honor this simple request, a relationship class might be in order. There's nothing wrong with asking for a little peace and quiet, a little time to yourself to regroup, especially when you are not feeling well.

Around here, we use words like…

I'm feeling fragile today.

I can't handle any new information today.

I'm having a bad day.

I'm having a sad day.

Whatever you say or do today will be wrong, so it's best to steer clear of me today.

It's not personal.

It's not you.

All I want is chocolate.

Let's go out to eat.

I can't stay awake today.

I think I'll just read a book for a while.

I can't seem to hold onto my thoughts today.

And when all else fails, I call an end to my day and go to bed. As Scarlett said, tomorrow is another day. So when your PMDD-ing woman goes to bed, consider that it might be to protect what she loves the most; you, and her family.

Chapter Nine

———•———

More Reader Comments

—·—

These are in regard to my blog post It's Not Personal, It's Just Your PMDD. Any responses from me are in italics.

—·—

This is SUCH good advice! Thank you for continuing to give encouragement and suggestions for how to help, other than pushing meds that do exactly what you said - create side effects to add onto the stress one is already dealing with! If anyone has an iPhone, I would highly recommend the P tracker. I've dealt with PMDD for almost 6 years now and until now never tracked my symptoms, I just know when my "off" days are going to be and when I'm most likely to have an episode. But with this app, you can chart your symptoms and write notes—help yourself remember what is going on around you. It's a great tool!!!

~.¼.~

Oh, but this is so true. The "what's the matter with you?" question is like a red flag to a bull, because, let's face it, how many days of the month do you accommodate the people around you, mood swings, demands, stresses and all, before your hormones dictate that you take care of "you" and snap?

~.¼.~

This post comes at an apt time. Was met with "I know you feel like crap, but you don't need to be mean to me, you're not even trying today, I want to hear that you're trying."

~.¼.~

This, my PMDD friends, is emotional manipulation. The partner is asking for something the woman is clearly not capable of giving at that moment. He speaks to her as if he is training a dog. And below, she first accepts the blame for his behavior, then realizes she is not entirely at fault here. Yay, you!

~.¼.~

I was trying SO hard it was a tough day and my 'reaction' was VERY minor in the grand scheme of things. But then I realized later he was bringing his own frustrations with him because of other circumstances. It's not always you...other people have tough days too.

~.¼.~

I want to thank you for bringing rationality to

something that is so inherently irrational. For the past two years, I've been coping with the realization that my life-long "insanity" is PMDD. All this time, I've been single. Now, I've met someone new and have not yet told him the "evil truth." Your blog is fantastic and really helps me to understand how to approach my new situation with this someone special. Thank you.

-\'/-

I am for sure bookmarking your site. I have been living with this since I was 11 years old. It gets worse when my life tends to be more stressful. I am just beginning to learn about PMDD. I believe I was mistakenly diagnosed with depression when I was 12 and mistakenly diagnosed with PCOS in my 20's. *[Polycystic Ovarian Syndrome]* I am now 33 and have had to have physical therapy for stress-related pain. It's all related to PMDD.

-\'/-

I've spent the last 4 hours crying off and on and arguing with my boyfriend while trying to explain to him that I just needed someone to talk to. PMDD is such a lonely disorder. Its rarity coupled with its extreme nature make it so difficult to cope with at times. I can't just talk to other women because in reality most of them haven't experienced this. My boyfriend keeps comparing it to PMS and he tries to make me feel better by saying all women go through it, but he is completely off base and misinformed. It is not PMS and most women don't go through this.

-\'/-

The thing I struggle with the most in my relationships is trying to convince people that I'm aware of my symptoms, but I can't control them. I can't simply will it all away. I have actually chosen to take an anti-anxiety drug during the luteal phase of my menstrual cycle. I have downloaded the WomanLog [calendar Android] app on my phone that helps me track my cycle. The drug helps tremendously, but since I only take them 2 weeks out of every month, I always have to wait 48 hours from taking the first pill for them to kick in with relief.

～✦～

If you are already tracking your cycle, and know when your period will arrive, why not start taking your anti-anxiety meds a day or two sooner? Don't wait for the symptoms to present themselves. Head them off at the pass!

～✦～

Prior to my diagnosis and treatment I attempted suicide once and threatened suicide at least 4 other times.

～✦～

I am embarrassed to admit that I have this illness to anyone as only two people in my life know that I suffer...my mom and my boyfriend. My mom is very supportive, but my boyfriend treats me like I am weak-minded. I'm not sure our relationship will survive this.

～✦～

I'm afraid to date anyone else for fear that no one will ever accept this about me.

～✦～

You need to go back to chapter one and work on acceptance of yourself.

＿ﾊﾞ＿

I feel hopeful at least that if I can encourage my boyfriend to become educated about what I am experiencing and how to better support me, then perhaps we can make it. I pray that one day he will realize when it comes to my PMDD, I don't want his opinion, I just want his love and support.

＿ﾊﾞ＿

I have been suffering from PMDD for what seems 3 years after beginning birth control. Once I stopped birth control last year, it has been a roller coaster as the monthly mood swings have been amped to full extent. I am screaming like a banshee, crying, throwing things, etc. and I can honestly say I sit back as if paralyzed and [horrified] in my own mind, trying to break free from the cycle of Jekyll and Hyde.

＿ﾊﾞ＿

I usually like things neat and in order (kind of a perfectionist) on a normal basis and it seems it becomes tenfold when I am in the PMDD zone. I want everything to be finished properly, no loose ends, or else.

＿ﾊﾞ＿

PMDD truly puts much stress on our relationship. My boyfriend is usually sweet and apologetic, trying to solve things before they get out of control and I, of course, want things to go my way. If they don't, hell will literally break loose. Sometimes I don't even feel it coming on and I will just turn into a ball of negativity and I can`t seem to tell myself to stop. It is as if I am in a trance, and

everyone around me has the problem (I know, clearly the PMDD talking).

~⅟~

I used to be a perfectionist, too, and while still working a full time job, would think everyone else was completely inept during my monthly time. How could I be surrounded by such pervasive incompetence and inefficiency? The world was filled with idiots. On my PMDD days, it still is.

Chapter Ten

---·---

Finding the Right Partner

Relationships and PMDD - Finding the Right Partner

Okay, now we're going to get into what I had in mind when I first thought about writing about PMDD and relationships. But then I realized that for any of us to have a successful relationship, we have to start with ourselves. We have to know ourselves, like ourselves, and be friends with ourselves before we can **successfully** have any sort of relationship with anyone else, be it a friendship, a family relationship, or a relationship with a significant other.

You can have all kinds of relationships with all kinds of people, but how many of them are truly successful? How many of them make you smile instead of sigh or groan? How many would you rather not have?

If you haven't thought about it, then take some time out now to do so. Pull out a pad of paper and pencil and divide a page into two columns. Now think about someone, and put their name in one column or the other. You can break the two columns into sub headings, if you like, such as:

1. Who lifts your spirit, and who tries to kill it?

2. Who treats you with the respect and dignity you deserve, and who ignores and steamrolls over you?

3. Who takes care of you, and who takes away from you? (I'm not just talking about time, energy, and money. I'm talking who are your emotional vampires?)

4. Who would drain you dry if you'd let them (and probably already has, several times over).

5. Who cheers you on as you go through life, and who drags you down?

6. Who is there for you, and who is not?

7. Who would you choose as a friend if you had to start all over again?

I would include relatives on this last designation, because you can also be friends with various relatives.

This last list, sad to say, also includes your partner or spouse. Some people are married to people they don't like, and would never choose as friends. What does that say about the state of these relationships?

In short, who treats you like you matter to them, and who doesn't?

But before you go pointing fingers, remember this: People will only treat you as well as you treat yourself. So if you don't treat yourself well, don't expect anyone else to. And if you don't make your boundaries clear, as to what you will and will not do or accept, there is no way people can respect those boundaries. People are not mind readers.

How do you know what your boundaries are? You take the time to get to know yourself, your likes and dislikes, tastes and preferences, and what you will and will not tolerate. If you don't know yourself in this way, or don't understand yourself at all, how can you explain your PMDD to anyone else? And if you don't treat yourself with dignity, respect, kindness, care, and consideration, how can you expect anyone else to?

Face it, most of us treat friends better than we do ourselves. We're there for friends, but when it comes to being there for ourselves, for any number of reasons we drop the ball. Why? Is it because we expect people to return the favors we do for them? To return the support and friendship we give them? Or do we expect our friends and family to "just know" when we need help and drop everything to lend a hand, like we do to them?

Dream on, ladies. Dream on.

Many of us are already in relationships, and have children. Children who depend on us to be there for them, no matter what kind of day we are having. Taking care of ourselves, seeing to our own wellness, helps us to be better able to take care of them. When we're calm, relaxed, rested, and happy, we're much better able to weather the storms life blows into our days—and provide that emotional stability our children need to grow into happy, well-adjusted adults.

They can't do that if we're in a bad relationship, whatever the reason. So if you're not willing to put forth the effort to find or create a healthy, stable, and supportive relationship for yourself, then do it for them—the kids who are counting on you to show them how life works. If you don't show them…who will?

To have a good relationship, you need a supportive partner. Period. If your partner isn't supportive of your needs as a woman with PMDD, you might as well be a salmon swimming upstream. But for your partner to be supportive of those needs, you have to know what those needs are. When you're having an episode, do you need calm and quiet, or do you need to be held? Do you need to be left alone, or do you want someone who can help to ease you out of your negative mood? Will flowers and candy help? Do you just want to watch TV or read a book, or do you want to talk?

The answers are as varied as can be. But the key to any good relationship is communication. Maybe one month you'll want to go out to dinner. Maybe another you'll want to take a long bath. Maybe you'll want to make some popcorn and watch a comedy. Maybe you'll want to go for a walk. Maybe you'll need a nap. Maybe you just want to feel appreciated.

Whatever you want, you need to be able to communicate that to your partner *during your non-PMDD times,* so they know what to do when you are in the PMDD zone. And if your partner won't cooperate…is he or she the right partner for you?

Never stay in a relationship because you are afraid no one else will want you. That's the PMDD talking. PMDD is a bully. And if it's your partner telling you no one else will want you, he or she is being a bully. Either way, PMDD or partner, it's abuse and not true.

Once you know what your pattern is, you need to let your partner know when your bad days are coming, and ask for some extra consideration on those days. If you have a really good relationship with your partner, he or she might be able to see the storm coming before it arrives. Years ago, there were many times I was completely unaware that I was starting to act out of character, until a good friend pointed it out. Then I had to decide if he was right or not, because nobody knows my mental, emotional, or physical state as well as I do.

Sometimes my friend was right, and sometimes he was wrong. When he was right, we'd go into PMDD mode. When he was wrong, I would do my best to figure out what was really bothering me, and if he was involved, we would talk about it. If he wasn't, we either dropped the subject—because I like to figure things out on my own, and he knows that about me—or I would ask for help in how to deal with the person or situation causing my anger and/or tears.

Beware of partners who tell you that you must be having an episode because you're upset with them for one reason or another. There are times in *everyone's* lives when we are genuinely angry or upset with someone about something. And that's okay. Anger and emotional upset are normal emotions and natural signals that something is not going right in our lives. They're like warning lights, flashing to let us know that "something is going on here" that needs to be addressed.

The key is to know the difference—are you genuinely angry, or has your PMDD kicked in?

If your PMDD has kicked in, revert to the list of code phrases I mentioned in chapter eight. What works with children and family members works as well with partners. Or make up your own list. Agree on your PMDD code phrases beforehand, when you are feeling healthy and well. Then, when the bad days come, you will be prepared and will have them ready to diffuse tense situations that arise.

A good relationship of any kind is based on mutual admiration and respect. If you're in a good relationship, your partner will respect your need for space or extra help or attention when the bad days come. If you're not, you will likely find yourself with a partner who ignores you, demeans you, eggs you on, refuses to believe you, and/or abandons you when you most need love and support. Partners like this only add to the problem, because they create stress. Stress exacerbates PMDD, so yes, your home environment does have a huge impact on your PMDD and ability to reach wellness.

The absolute, positive best thing you can do for yourself is to find a partner *who will not add to your stress* when you are already stressed. If your partner won't listen, then there is more going on in your relationship than your PMDD. Never let anyone blame you or your PMDD solely for the failures in a relationship, be they friends, family, or your significant other. As I have said many times over, it takes two to make a relationship, and two to break it. If you're trying, and the other party isn't— it's not just about your PMDD. They are using your PMDD as an excuse to avoid looking at whatever else may be going wrong in the relationship. On the flip side of that, you need to consider whether you are using your PMDD as a steam valve for what is going wrong in your relationship.

Sometimes PMDD can be made the scapegoat, as well. By

both parties.

So remember, PMDD is an explanation, not an excuse. Not for you, and not for anyone else. Do not let yourself or anyone else use your PMDD as an excuse to explain away bad behavior, on your part, or theirs. That only hurts the relationship, and keeps you from finding wellness.

If somebody loves you, truly loves you, they will work with you to find a way to make your life easier and your PMDD more bearable. They will be open to information and resources on the subject, and will want to help you get better. They will not walk away, refuse to help you, refuse to listen to you, and they will not cast 100% of the blame on you. They may not be happy with you at times, but they will be there for you.

If they are not…you need to start at the beginning of this book…and learn how to be there for yourself.

Chapter Eleven

———◆———

Advice for Partners of Women with PMDD

Dealing With PMDD - Advice for Men

I've spent quite a bit of time searching the internet for resources and advice for men dealing with a woman who suffers from PMDD. Unfortunately, most articles casually lump PMS and PMDD together, which does a great disservice to both women with PMDD and their partners. In the comment sections of these articles both men and women express anger and resentment toward women who experience true PMDD; the men claiming the articles give women a license to behave badly two weeks out of the month, and the women claiming the women with extreme mood swings give all women a bad name.

So, to clear a few things up…

20% of women suffer no pre-menstrual symptoms at all

80% of women suffer from some combination of pre-menstrual symptoms

20-40% experience moderate discomfort pre-menstrually

3-8% (possibly up to 10%) of menstruating women suffer from PMDD

This chapter is written for those who have partners with PMDD.

But before we get started, I want to say that whenever I read an article, report, or essay about PMDD, if the author lumps PMS and PMDD together as one, or describes PMDD as a "more extreme version of PMS," I view that entire document with skepticism. Because if they can't get that fundamental fact correct, then to me all information in that document is suspect.

And now, a quick primer on the differences between PMS and PMDD.

PMS deals primarily with physical symptoms. Bloating, aching, cramping, tenderness, fatigue, headaches, food cravings, and mild mood swings are the most well-known of the more than 150 symptoms possible. Some irritability, tension, sadness, weepiness, or any combination thereof is par for the course.

The major component of PMDD is mood swings in the extreme. PMDD affects your brain's capability to regulate itself, and therefore affects just about every other hormone in your body. That's not to say a woman with PMDD can't have bloating, aching, cramping, fatigue, cravings, and other physical symptoms. If she does, it may well be that she suffers from **both** PMDD **and** PMS, and once she gets her PMDD under control, all she'll be left with is some PMS.

Frankly, I think most women with PMDD would be

thrilled to simply suffer some form of PMS. Because PMS is to PMDD what a headache is to a migraine. There is a distinct difference, and that difference is *biological*—not mental. The biology of PMS and PMDD share many similarities, but at some point they split into completely different paths. An explanation of that is beyond the scope of this book.

For now, it's enough to know that PMS and PMDD are two completely different things.

That's not to say your relationship won't benefit from the advice presented in this chapter if your partner simply has PMS. But to make things clear: I am not talking about dealing with PMS anywhere in this book. I am talking about dealing with PMDD.

1. **Both you and your partner should make notes on a calendar or use some sort of app to make you aware of when she is most likely to be pre-menstrual.** This can be hard if her cycle is not regular, or she is approaching menopause, but do the best you can to identify patterns. An explanation of my pattern is provided in Flashback #2 in this book, A Perfect Storm of PMDD, and can give you an idea of what symptoms to look for.

Period Tracker is one app I have heard recommended several times. WomanLog is another. There are also several period tracking apps available specifically for men, but I would avoid those that treat a woman's cycle as if it's a joke. You know, the ones that tell you when to run for the hills. Running away from a relationship never solved anything.

On the flip side, if your partner is in denial, and claims there's nothing wrong with her—track her cycle separately. In many cases, the man can tell before the woman that she's entering her pre-menstrual phase, because he's watching from the outside, while—either consciously or sub-consciously— she's distracted by trying to cope with (deny, suppress, compensate for) the unwanted changes going on in her brain and body.

Please note: There are women who are in complete denial that anything different is happening to them, and then there are women who know what's happening, but "don't want to deal with this right now" because they are too busy to, and so they pretend nothing is happening, and that they aren't feeling any differently than usual—until it's too late to do anything about it, and the episode erupts full force.

Determine which type of woman you live with, and keep track accordingly.

2. **If she's indicated that this is what she would prefer, try to stay clear of her until the episode passes.** This has nothing to do with you, or her love for you. It's due to her heightened sensitivity to any combination of the five senses. She literally can't handle any more sensory input—be it bright lights, loud noises, touch of any kind, strong smells, or even certain foods. If a woman with PMDD has allergies, they can be exacerbated pre-menstrually. If she has any other condition, such as arthritis, diabetes, lupus, or fibromyalgia, those can be exacerbated as well.

Even if she's otherwise healthy, during an episode of PMDD a woman is literally a walking bundle of nerves. Unfortunately for both of you, this heightened sensitivity and very real discomfort can be so distracting that it makes her unable to focus on things like questions, requests, conversations, or simple instructions. (Now you know why she forgot to put coffee in the coffeemaker when she made coffee.)

Take the first one, for example: You have a question that requires some thought and consideration.

Examples would be:

Major purchases—house, car, appliances, maybe that boat, motorcycle, or sportscar you've always wanted (not a good time to bring it up)

Health decisions

Financial decisions

Employment decisions

Decisions involving having or raising children

Vacation plans

Any change of routine or structure in your life

Why? Because during a PMDD episode a woman's brain is not functioning properly. This has nothing to do with how intelligent she is. This is her brain chemistry being disrupted due to the hormonal shifts taking place in her body. During a PMDD episode it can take all of her concentration simply to focus on the basics of getting through each day. If you come at her with anything resembling a major decision, it could overload her brain and cause a meltdown.

So if she asks for space during that time, please give it to her.

3. **Be patient.** Dealing with anybody on a short fuse can be challenging. If she snaps at you, or does something that irritates you, don't lose your temper and fight back. It won't do any good, and in most cases will only make things worse. Just (discreetly) take a deep breath, maybe say a prayer, and ignore

whatever she just did that bothered you. Remember that she's not normally like this and she'll be herself again soon.

4. **Do not enable immature or abusive behavior.** I've said all along, *PMDD is an explanation, not an excuse.* Being emotional does not excuse inappropriate behavior, any more than being drunk excuses offensive behavior. If she's being immature, yelling, shouting, stomping, snapping, cursing, slamming or throwing things, don't respond with your own immature behavior. She at least has an explanation for it—a biological explanation. What's yours?

Stay calm and leave the room if you have to, until she settles down. Let her know you'll be nearby, but you can't have a conversation with her when she's upset like this. Believe me, she knows she's being irrational. But without conscious effort at awareness, she can't stop herself any more than she could stop an allergic reaction. If you calmly say you'll be happy to continue this conversation when she's feeling better, things will settle down a lot more quickly than if you respond with your own emotional outburst. In my original blog post on this same subject I suggested pointing out to her that she's being irrational or immature, but I have since abandoned that idea. Telling people who are behaving irrationally that they are being irrational does not add to the conversation. It only frustrates and angers them more. So walk away. Simply refuse to engage.

5. **As long as she's behaving like an adult, listen to her, even if she's not making any sense.** Try to figure out what the REAL problem is. If she's complaining about something that's never bothered her before, or doesn't usually bother her, most likely what she's saying is "I feel miserable, and there's

nothing I can do about it, so I'm looking for something else to change and hoping that will make me feel better." This is a time of true desperation for her. She's looking for *anything,* rational or irrational, that will make her feel better. This is a good time to suggest she take some time out for herself, maybe a hot bath, or a cup of tea and a good book, or whatever soothes her soul. Let her know you support her need to have a little time to pamper herself in whatever way makes her the happiest.

But beware of sending her out on a shopping spree. Retail therapy will only make things much, much worse when the mood has passed and the bills come in.

6. **Don't take it personally.** During an episode of PMDD, you can count on her emotions getting the best of her, and she'll probably question your relationship. She might question you. Might question her whole life and everything she believes or stands for. This is normal and natural for a woman during an episode of PMDD. As mentioned in Number 5, she's feeling helpless, and sometimes when people feel helpless they look for other things they can control, and that might mean bringing up topics or suggesting changes that trigger *your* emotions. It's like some deep, dark part of her wants to push *your* buttons, set off *your* triggers, make *you* feel as out of control as she does.

I call this the PMDD brain, the brain that takes over when you are in full-fledged PMDD crisis mode, and yes, it can and will bait you if given half a chance. The PMDD brain is reptilian in its desire to destroy any and all obstacles in its path, including her, you, your family, your relationship, and anything near and dear to either one of you. Think *The Terminator,* or any one of those movies rife with robotic killers.

It's not just you the PMDD brain seeks to destroy. It's her, too. From the inside.

Can you even begin to *imagine* what that feels like? Your own brain seeks to destroy you? Fifteen percent of women with PMDD who attempt suicide succeed. God only knows how many more contemplate killing themselves every single month, but from the volume of posts on the subject in several public forums, it happens a lot.

Truly, your best defense against her PMDD brain is to stay level-headed and calmly say, "Okay, I understand." What you understand is that you're still the same person she loved before her PMDD episode kicked in, and her change in perception of you and her life overall is the PMDD talking, not her. It's almost as if you are slowly raising your hands in the air and saying, "I don't want any trouble," to someone who has taken your partner hostage. Just like she needs to separate herself from her PMDD, you need to realize that this destructive behavior is coming not from her, the woman you love, but from an entity inside her. Fighting her, fighting *it,* by whatever name you want to call her PMDD, can only end badly for both of you.

7. **Be compassionate.** Think about a time when stress or physical changes made you hard to get along with. Have you ever been sleep-deprived? Maybe you had an accident or were in the hospital, and the chronic pain made you want to lash out at everybody. Again, put yourself in her shoes. Not only is she experiencing uncomfortable physical symptoms, but her hormones also ebbing and flowing, making it almost impossible for her to know from one moment to the next how she feels or what she wants. Then her fight or flight reptilian PMDD brain

kicks in.

Think of the effect testosterone has had on you, like when you get sexually aroused, or on any occasion when you felt aggression or rage. You remember how you felt caught up in the emotion, caught up in the moment, how it made you want to say and do things you ordinarily wouldn't say or do?

That's what's happening to her.

Again, her PMDD brain is primed to win at all costs, no matter who or what is destroyed in the process. To *her* brain, this irrational argument about who walked the dog or took out the trash the last time *is* life or death.

That's how skewed PMDD makes our thought processes. We see every crumb of dissent as a full frontal attack on everything we think and believe. PET scans of a woman's brain during PMDD shows the same configuration as that of a combat veteran with PTSD.

This is real, folks, with no easy solutions.

8. **Be forgiving and reassuring—but not patronizing.** Her insecurities will definitely come up during an episode of PMDD, and with her heightened sensitivity, and her PMDD brain serving as a bully, every negative thought she has will be magnified ten times over. If she doesn't consciously stop the negative thoughts, they will flow through her mind in an endless loop of lies.

Can you imagine your own brain lying to you repeatedly? All day long?

If you can get her to talk about her thoughts, fine. Some women won't want to, because they know the thoughts are irrational, even while they are having them. They just don't know how to stop them. Nobody wants to share irrational thoughts, and then remember the irrational things they said when the episode is over. When the episode is over, it's OVER. She wants to get on with putting her life back on track.

If she feels unloved and insecure, she'll probably act out, which will make you not want to be around her, which her brain will tell her "confirms" her negative thoughts. Most women feel insecure about their bodies to start with, maybe even their lovemaking, child-rearing, housekeeping, creative or professional skills, and if they're in any way insecure about *your* feelings for them, this is when that insecurity will come out.

So try to give her a few extra compliments (and don't be offended if she doesn't believe you, or snaps at you for it), and—if she'll let you (remember those heightened sensory sensitivities)—be more affectionate. If she won't let you near her, don't make her feel badly by taking it personally. Deep inside, she wants you there, by her side, fighting this bully in her brain with her. But her PMDD brain knows that, and won't allow her to show any vulnerability or weakness to its enemy.

Guilt is the last thing a woman with PMDD needs when she's feeling unlovable. Tell her you understand and you'll be around if she changes her mind.

That could well be all it takes to melt her defenses.

Chapter Twelve

———◆———

Even More Comments from Readers

We're just under halfway through the book now, so I thought you might appreciate an opportunity to learn about the tragedy that is PMDD as it is reflected in relationships overall. There is no doubt in my mind that you will recognize yourself and your situation in the comments that follow. If nothing else, you can take heart in the fact that you are not alone.

More so than the other comment sections, this one contains comments from both men and women. Again, any responses from me are written in italics. There is no requirement to read this chapter. I have included it only to show you there are two sides to this debilitating disorder. On a side note, based on what you have read in this book so far, you may now be able to tell which of the following relationships will succeed—and which ones will not.

⋅⋅⋅

I have read so many things on PMDD and nothing has ever been more correct than this... I will be showing this to my boyfriend...Thank you.

～✳～

What this means is you must look to many aspects of your lifestyle to really be rid of PMDD. You must focus on your physical health, your mental and emotional health, your spiritual well-being if you will, and your social health as well! This sounds like quite a lot, but in reality you can make a lot of small changes to your life bit by bit, and start seeing dramatic improvement of your PMDD.

～✳～

We got engaged after she left me on one occasion and we were set to get married. The accusations continued and basically there was no consistency in the relationship. It was like an emotional rollercoaster. It did not make sense. Anyway, we didn't get married as it became so stressful ... She was literally all over the place, coming and going, moving in and out, it was absolute chaos. I couldn't believe what was happening every month. My work suffered as I couldn't sleep and I lost my job, got another one, and then lost that as well, due to not being able to focus on it.

～✳～

The advice here is good, but not always easy to keep a level head about. I *think* this is what we're dealing with, but it always becomes the worst about a week AFTER the PMS part... which means it sneaks up on her quite frequently, and I don't always have the energy or patience to deal with it.

─ⁿⁱ─

I'm just worn down with being the target every month.

─ⁿⁱ─

The worst part of it is the uncertainty. I know that at some point my wife is going to change and project a thousand negative emotions right into my head, then be as calm and as normal and loving as the girl I fell in love with, but with no acknowledgment of the turmoil that just ripped straight through the heart of our relationship.

─ⁿⁱ─

Daily I work professionally negotiating with aggressive, overly emotional and irrational people, but nothing compares to the frustration and hatred that can flare up when I find myself drawn into one of my wife's episodes. Losing track of her cycle is the dumbest thing I can do. I have a calendar with everything PMDD related written in code…Just in case.

─ⁿⁱ─

I won't sugar coat it with positive think. It's a hard path to choose, and after a few years of focused learning, tracking her cycle, watching for triggers, evaluating what works and what doesn't, you then have to learn how to control **yourself** as well as your wife's environment every half cycle.

─ⁿⁱ─

It's VERY HARD to get any man to do all the above; they simply do not understand. Even when I explain it, he

still does things to worsen the condition. He's told me if I keep up with this every month, he will leave me.

~ᴗ~

I am only 24 and think I have PMDD to the extreme level. I have suffered ever since i started my period and it has caused me to destroy so much of my life (the bits i love most)!!! now after being in a relationship for 8 years and only just realizing this is what I have it is very comforting to think i can help my partner!!!

~ᴗ~

It's easy to say "It's not her fault," or "She can't help it." But being emotionally, verbally and physically abused by a woman with PMDD Is STILL abuse! Do NOT tolerate it! Yes, make a decent effort to suggest help. I would suggest video recording all PMDD episodes. Do so for a few months. Then show her how BAD her behavior is. Do it in a counseling session preferably. DO NOT TOLERATE ABUSE!

~ᴗ~

As a person who has captured their PMDD gf on film and showed her the results. I HIGHLY discourage that. An explanation of the behavior while she is calm and rational with no PMDD episode works the best. A video will just ignite depression and anger.

~ᴗ~

I am so overwhelmed. I have been married for almost two years and have only recently been informed that the reason for the now apparent monthly crisis we have

endured was due to PMDD. We are a day or two into what appears to be this month's cycle and already I am being verbally assassinated and demeaned in it seems every possible way. She will cut me down badly and demand an apology if my reaction isn't loving. Her focus will remain on demanding an apology (even if one is not due) while continuing to be degrading for days.

~*~

I am trying to understand how she must be feeling. It's difficult when she claims she gets along fine with everyone from work and her family and that it is just me. She has made some progress as she is the one who shared this cause with me. I asked her if this was the week but she denied it. In the beginning she was physically attacking and caused noticeable dental damage. She attempted suicide almost two years ago as well.

~*~

I am frustrated that I am not doing good at handling her incredible mean statements as I have some hope that if this diagnosis is accurate that she may not mean all these terrible things even though they seem convincing.

~*~

I have had this and far worse for much longer. When PMDD takes over she will try to destroy you with words and deeds. It seems to be evil personified. But when I have looked into my wife's eyes the terrifying - yet somehow reassuring thing - was that this clearly was not the love of my life raging before me but a completely different person. The real woman was - is - the wonderful person that graces my life in between these nightmarish descents into sheer and utter hell.

～ン～

It has been an ongoing and bruising battle all through the years. The children are a real blessing. They have had a rough time but know that their mother is wonderful when she is not transformed into something frightening by PMDD.

～ン～

I've been going through this for 3 years now. The only way I can describe it is Ground Hog Day from hell. The way she looks at me, the stabbing words. I've only recently learned of this disorder, I didn't know what was going on every month. I'm happy to have this info, because at least I can see I'm not alone and as hard as it is to believe during an episode, it's not her fault. It's so hard not to take it personal when she is so cold and vicious. I just don't know if I have the strength to go through this hell every month for the rest of my life. But, when the episode ends and she is back I fall in love with her all over again. I'm so lost at what to do.

～ン～

My wife and i have been married for 12 years, and this started 18 months ago out of nowhere 6 months after our son was born. All these stories are what's happening to us. PMDD has stolen my wife, and our lives. She is deep in denial, but after showing her these and other stories i hope she gets it. We have been in an episode for 15 days now, this is the longest lasting one. Probably because her period is over a week late. it feels like i am fighting for my

life, and the pure hatred towards me is harsh. When she gets her period this all goes away and we have a week of normal till it starts again.

~ン~

I've been married for 18 years and I recall hints of PMDD every so often for the first 13 years but the past five years have been a powder keg of anger and violent profanity-laced one-sided arguments. I and my oldest daughter wondered where is this coming from. I took the blame for the outbursts, thinking it was something I said or did, but my daughter said, "Dad, you're not doing anything to cause this." And the more I tried to make sense of the monthly train wreck that is my wife the more nuts and angry I got. Then I noticed there was a pattern or a cycle to these episodes. She became indifferent, angry, irrational, emotional, destructive, and physically abusive. She denies there is a problem and if I persist she snaps so I ease off and tell the kids to steer clear of mom when she seems angry. Divorce has crossed my mind but the saving graces are our beautiful kids. They deserve a mom, a dad, and a home.

~ン~

I have been in and out of a relationship with the same wonderful woman for three years. She has broken up with me anywhere from 7-9 times. It is absolutely predictable. The break ups are inexplicable and all happen right before her period. During or after her period she loves me again and wants to get back together with me...anywhere from two to five days after we break up we are back together.

~ン~

I've been reading various PMDD websites for the last 3 years and have heard lots of stories that have helped me. From a man's perspective, this is seriously tough. After about 4 months together (seeing each other twice a week) I started to notice things I didn't understand. I'd get accused of things that I hadn't done, like fancying other women, and I would spend hours defending myself to her. She would regularly say inappropriate things. She'd storm off and regularly misinterpret things I said. I would always beg her to come back and I would apologize to keep the peace.

It takes everything i have to suppress it at work and it does come out... I've lost two jobs in my life due to PMDD. I've ruined more relationships with bfs and friends though... And yes i notice i come home and unleash it and i feel like a piece of crap after... I will show this article to my bf. He doesn't believe me on any of it and just says i'm crazy and need help... That makes me very angry and when he responds to my outbursts negatively it makes it hard....

I love this girl so much and she is incredible. Beautiful, funny, intelligent. Everything. Unfortunately she has left me for good now it seems because we weren't making any progress and she is now allegedly with someone else. I'm heartbroken but need to focus on getting my life back together. I've contemplated finishing my life over this as I couldn't bear being without her. I've been to counseling myself because I couldn't understand why it wasn't working and it has created some issues with me.

As I have been dealing with the same nightmare for many years, I envy the young men who are not so engulfed in the NEVER ENDING NIGHTMARE. I will not leave my wife, however I am doomed to hell on earth. Mine will not seek help. She is killing us both. Those of us on the target end of this horror surprise epic have limits on what our mind can withstand. Go for a real life, and never look back!

So true! And though I wouldn't leave my wife for anything, I couldn't agree more. If you are with someone and have noted they exhibit this behavior, my advice is to run before you are completely engulfed. Seriously, you are looking at relatively good odds of being miserable for half of the rest of your days.

For me and apparently many other men, it's much too late to turn back now.

I do want to point out that PMDD does end with menopause (when a woman stops having her period), but if left untreated, her PMDD will get a LOT worse before it gets better, especially during the years leading up to menopause, and will leave her prone to Major Depressive Disorder in her post menopausal—or so called "golden" years. Not much to look forward to, which is why I heartily recommend doing everything possible to get a handle on her PMDD before perimenopause sets in.

―⁂―

I have been seeking treatment for years! My issue is, there is none. Antidepressants might help a tiny bit but they also rob you of your "normal time." That is, making you feel very blah when you could actually be feeling like a normal, sane person. My PMDD is so obvious and physical, I can feel it arrive and I can feel it leave. It is sudden and stays for 10 days! It is horrible. People like to think I am making it up or exaggerating. That just makes the problem worse.

―⁂―

My wife is in total denial that she has any problem. I have been away from home for almost two months now. She said she was out of denial two months ago, but then slipped away again. Now she says she doesn't want me back because I made up this illness. We talk on the phone and she says she loves me, and wants to talk to me and everything is good for a few days. Then she starts getting distant, and starts to ignore me. I know her period is due any day now so I'm hoping she pops out of it this time. She missed her period in July and finally got it mid-August, but we had a huge blowout at that time. Maybe that was the reason for her not asking me to come home that time. When we talk on the phone she cries almost the whole time, she says she wants to be with me, but she is confused.

―⁂―

She is confused because her true self wants to be with you, but her reptilian PMDD brain is taking no prisoners. Seriously, you cannot imagine how hard a woman with PMDD must fight her very own brain when it is trying to destroy everything she loves. Sometimes she wins, but most of the time, she does not. And everyone involved suffers for it.

‑‑‑‑‑

I think I have PMDD. I just realized that every month for a couple of days I feel very irritable, I even rage and normally I am a very calm person. I feel like quitting my job and I question every single aspect of my life. Last week I put my relationship at risk because I behaved very badly with my bf. I embarrassed him in front of his friends and on our way home I screamed, I hit him, and I told him he could walk away from me.

‑‑‑‑‑

My girlfriend and I have been dating for 3 years, she is 42 yrs old, and I believe she has SEVERE PMDD. She takes Zoloft and double doses a week before (when she doesn't forget) and can't take BC due to past reactions. Last weekend I went over to her place (one week before her period was due) and stayed the weekend...she worked Sunday but I made dinner and cleaned her house (which was a mess) before she got home. We watched a movie and I would say had a fair evening...She is usually distant and cold during her episodes...She's very affectionate when she is not. The next 2 days she was off from work so on her last day off via text I said I was going to come down and she said, "Well, what if I have plans?" I asked, do you? She said no. Mind you, this is never an issue... I recognized right away I was being baited for a fight... (In the most caring and understanding way possible) I said, "I can come visit on a different day."

But she hung up on me.

~⅏~

I have been reading blogs for men who deal with this and it helps a lot...we all are dealing with EXACTLY the same women. Everyone seems as stressed as I am...some of the stories are even a little funny...because I identify with the anger and sheer resentment she treats me with during these times. The worst part for me is being ignored, sent to voicemail, sending a text and getting no response, etc. She has a high pressure job that she excels at and I can't help but resent her clients that see and speak to her more than I do during her episodes.

~⅏~

I love this man profoundly. I want to marry him!!!! He is very disappointed (I can tell). I even had suicidal thoughts. I am going to look for help but I have to do it by myself because he'll believe that I'm trying to give excuses. I take care of my relationships and my job like precious diamonds and then one day I wake up and I want to destroy everything... And the worst is the guilt and shame afterward.

~⅏~

I have cried my eyes out. She would and will not look into the matter. It has only become worse. Now I am "single" again after 20 years. I miss her ....

~⅏~

Brother, if it has gone that long with her in denial, refusing to seek therapy or help, and disregarding what she has done to you, then you are better off this way. I know it may not seem that way at the moment, but stay strong and determined and focus on always moving forward and relearning how to take care of yourself. I'm in the same boat as you, my wonderful (sometimes, and deep down always) wife of 8 years will become my ex-wife this week. As much as I long to show her these sites, with the hopes of happily-ever-after, the one thing I keep coming back to is I can and will sit down and talk about her [PMDD] and textbook BPD *[Bipolar Disorder],* but not until the divorce papers are signed and final. If something miraculous happens subsequent to that, so be it. Otherwise, with absolute certainty, I will be better off and lead a much happier, fulfilling life whether alone or with somebody else. It hurts now and that will continue for a while, nothing you can do about it other than refuse to let it stop you from living your life. It, and you, will get better with time and distance, and the hurt will diminish and come less often. The more you do for yourself emotionally, socially, and spiritually, will hasten the arrival of happiness, and better yet peace and contentment.

⋅⋊⋅

Keeping you, her, and everyone like us in my prayers.

Chapter Thirteen

———◆———

Tips for Partners Dealing with PMDD

Top 20 Tips for Partners Dealing with PMDD

Unfortunately, my research has uncovered a complete lack of serious information for men on the subject of PMDD, so here it is, short and sweet, a list of the top 20 things you can do for your partner with PMDD.

1. Believe her. When she tells you what she's experiencing, **believe** her. Even if it doesn't make sense. Because PMDD doesn't make sense. The symptoms are as unique and individual as the woman having them.

2. Do not tease her. Do not make fun of her, as this is a serious and often debilitating condition.

**3. Chart her symptoms daily, either together or on

your own. If she refuses to admit there's a problem, then do it on your own so that you can be prepared for when the storm hits.

4. Consult your chart or app when considering social events, activities, or vacations and such. Surprises and big decisions come under this heading, too.

5. Learn as much information as you can about PMDD from reliable resources. If they have a product to sell you, any type of product, proceed with caution.

6. Understand that if it is not treated, her PMDD will only get worse. It could end up as Major Depressive Disorder.

7. **Help her to find a doctor who will listen to her and help her.** This may take several tries, as most doctors are not trained in the treatment of PMDD. Traditionally trained medical doctors will only offer you birth control or antidepressants, since they are the only drugs medically approved for treatment of PMDD by the FDA. Your best bet is to find a naturopathic doctor or nurse practitioner.

8. Don't let her negative thoughts and feelings get the better of her—or you. If she shares them with you, gently remind her it's the PMDD talking, not her, and postpone any major discussions/decision making for a few days.

9. Be supportive and encouraging as she tries different things to feel better. Make a note of what works and what doesn't. Share this with her doctor.

10. Help her to get enough rest. Sleep is when our bodies re-regulate themselves. If we don't have enough (sleep) time to do the work needed, we start the day at a disadvantage.

11. Join her for moderate exercise. Exercise is always

more fun with a friend. I have found a walk of 45 minutes can buy me up to two hours of PMDD-free time.

12. Encourage her to eat healthy. (Avoid alcohol, caffeine, sugar, sugar substitutes, energy drinks, anything made with high fructose corn syrup, and white rice and flour, for starters.)

13. Buy her some high quality dark chocolate. Keep it on hand for the bad days.

14. Do what you can to keep stressful situations to a minimum. PMDD feeds on stress.

15. Do not accept any behavior that is abusive. Ever.

16. Do not return such behavior if it happens. Calmly walk away and resume your conversation when she is more in control of herself. Be firm about refusing to engage when she is out of control or abusive. When she gets this way, the PMDD bully in her brain is in full control, and determined to destroy whatever it can.

17. Remember that she literally is not herself during an episode of PMDD. Try not to hold the things she says and does against her. It's not personal, and it's not about you. It's the bully egging her on.

18. Be as comforting as she will allow you to. If she won't let you near her, let her know you will be nearby if she needs you.

19. Don't expect her to be full of sunshine and laughter when she's not having a PMDD episode. A healthy, balanced, and emotionally well-rounded woman feels every emotion—not just the good ones.

20. Last, but not least: Do not blame every time she becomes irritated, annoyed, angry, afraid, or upset on her PMDD. Nothing is more irritating than having a genuine concern or grievance, and being told, "It's your PMDD again, isn't it?"

Maybe it is, and maybe it isn't. Take the time to check her chart to see if she's supposed to be having an episode, and then carefully sort through (usually by talking it out) and separate what is her PMDD and what is a genuine fear or concern on her part. Encourage her to feel and express the full range of emotions, just like people without PMDD do.

More than anything, a woman with PMDD just wants to feel normal. These 20 tips will go a long way toward helping your partner do just that.

～

More Tips For Those With Partners Who Have PMDD

The previous section, while it will go a long way toward stabilizing your relationship with a woman in the throes of a PMDD episode, was barely the tip of the iceberg. So here are some more tips and information on how to cope with your partner when she's feeling her worst.

Once again, most articles I've read were about how awful it is for the man, who has to deal with all sorts of aberrant behavior on the part of his partner. There doesn't seem to be much understanding or empathy for the woman actually going through the brain chemical changes over which she has no control.

Her responses to it, yes, she does have some control over those, depending on her level of self-awareness. But for the most part, her reptilian brain has taken over and is simply telling her to survive at all costs—with no thought for collateral damage.

So the first thing I want to re-emphasize is empathy. **Put yourself in her shoes,** and my guess is you'll discover you wouldn't want to have a body and brain you have no control over for several days a month. How would you feel if your thoughts—due to a biological disconnect between your brain and your mouth—came out of your mouth as something else entirely—something actually hurtful to those you love the most? How would you feel if no matter how hard you tried to eat right and/or stay in shape, your body suddenly just puffed up like a water balloon and wouldn't cooperate? What if it actually undermined all your best efforts by bringing on intense cravings for things you know you shouldn't eat, cravings for things that actually make your condition worse?

This isn't about her appetite, it's about her brain, screaming for fuel, for carbs, for glucose, and it doesn't care where or how she gets it. The PMDD brain is like a parasite, only it doesn't care if it kills its host. The PMDD brain does not reason. It cannot reason. And caught up in the middle of its insatiable demands is a woman who *knows* that what is happening is wrong, but does not know how to *stop* it.

How would you feel if for *up to half of each month,* nothing you thought or said or did made sense?

One article I read said women could be touchy—touchy!—about being labeled as a raving lunatic for a few days a month. As if the women involved had no business being so sensitive. It also said very few women will admit they're affected by PMDD. Would you feel comfortable telling people, "Oh, don't mind me, my mind just goes berserk every now and then?" Would you want the strange looks that come with such a statement, would you want people steering a wide path around you because you just admitted there's something not quite right about you? Would you want them declining to hire you or trying to take your children from you?

So don't try to be helpful (or antagonistic) by pointing out her PMDD symptoms. She's well aware of what she is feeling. Anxious, edgy, jittery, depressed, clumsy, fat, foolish, frightened, sleepy, weepy, ravenous, disorganized, out of control…the list goes on.

Even more important is that you don't use any of the above symptoms to goad her into a PMDD rage with sarcasm. We all know men deal with stress through humor. Even if she loves it on her good days, this is not the time to express that aspect of your personality.

Your best bet is to save your meant-to-be-funny comments and war stories for your buddies, and simply act like nothing out of the ordinary is happening at home. Help to make your partner feel as accepted and normal as possible.

This does not mean you have to accept any kind of behavior she throws at you. Abuse is abuse, whether your partner means it or not. Again, PMDD is an explanation, not an excuse, and you should never accept abusive behavior under any conditions.

I also can't say this enough: Don't spring any big surprises on her. Remember she's doing everything she can just to cope with her everyday life, to stay on an even keel in a body that is physically betraying her, and emotionally tilting her from one extreme to another. Her goal is to just get through the day, one step at a time, without being labeled crazy. Big news, big plans, big surprises can wait for a day when she's better equipped to handle them.

But if you forget: Never trust any big decisions made while she is under the influence of her PMDD. This includes decisions she may come to regarding your relationship. If she says she wants out...do what you can to stay calm, and wait until the storm passes. If when it does she still wants out...then you have a different problem, and she might really mean it.

Take it easy on social activities. If you felt like an acne factory or a beached whale and couldn't seem to control what you put in your mouth (or what popped out of it), would you want to go to a party? A food binge can be great fun, if that's what you want to be doing—if that's your way of celebrating good times or good news. But if you're watching your weight—and what woman isn't at one point or another?—taking her "food binge" show on the road is the last thing she wants to be doing.

The same goes for her emotional outbursts. It's hard enough to keep a lid on things at home. Do you really want to put her in a situation where she spends the evening either snarling at your friends and family or weeping at every misinterpreted comment? Because a PMDD brain will always focus on the negative, and even if you didn't say or mean anything negative at all, even if you compliment her, her brain is being flooded with negative thoughts and images, and eventually the dam will burst—putting a huge damper on your evening out.

And then she'll feel miserable about it. The misery comes from the woman, not from her PMDD brain. The PMDD brain is satisfied when she is miserable, because it has succeeded in its mission—ruining your (and her) day/plans/evening/event. Whether it did or did not, and whether the PMDD-ing woman admits it or not, she will always blame herself for anything that goes wrong during these dark periods of time in her cycle.

Be understanding of her cravings. Just as men do, women seek comfort food when they feel miserable. During a PMDD episode, a woman will especially seek carbs. Doing so is a natural way to boost the level of both glucose and serotonin in her body, and she knows this on a subconscious level. Where it gets confusing is the food and advertisement industries have done their best to convince us certain foods and drinks are healthy when they are not. So while on a very primitive level, your partner's body is craving something to make her feel better, what manifests is a desire to eat everything in sight in the hopes of finding that magic solution. Not to mention the reptilian brain is on the hunt for fuel and doesn't care where it comes from.

It's best to have good quality carbs already on hand for when these cravings strike. I find that whole wheat or multi-grain toast with no-added-sugar jam (but not the kind sweetened with artificial sweeteners instead of sugar), a bowl of whole or multi-grain cereal with organic milk, or a bit of good quality dark chocolate does the trick. When we consume large amounts of cheap chocolate candy we are looking for the same effect, but in the wrong place. The added calories from the sugar and fat that come along with the added amount of chocolate needed to reach the same serotonin boost as a good quality piece of dark chocolate only causes our PMDD symptoms to worsen. They also cause us to gain weight.

But sometimes, the woman's level of serotonin dips so low that nothing short of a pizza or plate of lasagna will do. If that's the case, then go for it guilt-free. You might even plan pizza or Italian night around her cycle, and see if that improves things.

Take on some of her workload. Whatever you can do to help out, do it with an attitude of love, not resentment. If she asks you to help around the house, do what she asks. If she wants you to run an errand, please do the same. The slightest bit of effort to appreciate what she's going through will go a long way toward soothing her, and is it really worth the effort to argue over who emptied the dishwasher last?

It's true that things that don't usually bother her will bother her greatly when she's having an episode. Just keep in mind who your real partner is, and go along with what she says. The sooner you do, the sooner her episode will pass. Why is this? I'm no scientist, but I think it has to do with her body releasing bonding hormones.

That's right, bonding hormones, oxytocin in particular. Google it. Stress (and the accompanying stress hormones) will prolong her episode. Oxytocin, (and the accompanying calming hormones), can bring a reprieve to the episode. So if you want the madness to end sooner, the best thing you can do is find a way to get her oxytocin flowing by doing what she asks, as long as it's a reasonable request.

If you're a mature adult, you know what reasonable and unreasonable is. We don't need to go into it here.

Treat her like you appreciate her. Every woman loves to be appreciated, no matter what mood she's in. During an episode of PMDD, with all those negative thoughts running an endless loop inside her head, your partner needs extra special care. Reassurance is always nice, but might not be believed or accepted. Understand that the negative thoughts in her brain are overwhelming the positive ones you're trying to get across. Be patient. Be persistent. Let her know you care, and you're there for her if she needs you. She'll meet you more than half way if she possibly can.

If she doesn't, it's because she can't, or doesn't understand enough about what's happening to her to stop the train of negative thoughts in her mind. It's not because she doesn't want to, or doesn't love you. (Unless she truly enjoys being a drama queen, and that is a different situation/condition/disorder altogether.)

It's not about you at all. Remember that, and don't take the negative things she says to you personally. In a few days time, the woman you love will return, and when she does, it would be a good time to discuss what may have gone wrong between the two of you during her most recent episode.

A lot of women will want to forget what happened, pretend it didn't happen at all, and that's quite normal, but not the best way to deal with it. Talking it out with your partner when she's feeling herself is the best way to prevent unwanted behaviors and situations in the future.

The Bible says it best: *Love is patient, love is kind. It does not* *envy, it does not boast, it is not proud. It is not rude, it is not self-seeking, it is not easily angered, it keeps no record of wrongs. Love does not delight in evil but rejoices with the truth. It always protects, always trusts, always hopes, always perseveres.* ~ 1 Corinthians 13

All a woman with PMDD is looking for is the same thing everyone wants—love and acceptance.

The strangest thing is, the more we accept, the less we'll have to. What we resist persists. So don't fight your partner's PMDD. Go with it, roll with it—and watch the storm waves grow smaller over time.

Chapter Fourteen

———◆———

Readers Speaking Out

Again, there is no obligation to read these, but they may help you to feel less alone. As always, any responses from me are in italics.

⇜

Your writing gives both hope and comfort, not to mention the advice is truly good and might save someone from this suffering.

⇜

Two thoughts:

1) Men suffer from PMDD too. I am considering seeking treatment for my developing distress/depression. I am not certain, but I think my body has learned to sense my wife's coming PMDD episode. I get depressed/irritable a day or two before PMDD sets in.

2) God bless those of you willing to stay and love your wife

with PMDD. The grace of a marital vow is key to this. I do not mean to be callous, but those of you who are saying "my girlfriend" might consider that since you have not yet made a promise "for better or for worse," you should seriously consider that this woman might be better off living a single life and being able to have the quiet, peaceful environment she needs to avoid exacerbating her PMDD each month.

PMDD can spiral downward if not treated. Medical treatment is iffy and getting the peace-and-quiet treatment is almost impossible with children. You, as a father, will one day conceive children. Strongly consider if you want your child to grow up with a mother who drives them through hell for a week or two EVERY month. Breaking up with your girlfriend and suffering that loss now might be the loving thing to do for the sake of the children you will conceive with a different woman, a wife that does not have such a grave, debilitating, and destructive (to others) disorder.

I look back at the warning signs during our courtship and know I could have saved her, my children, and myself much suffering. I thank God, however, for the grace of the Sacrament of Marriage that carries us all through the suffering as we share in the Cross of Christ. I know that, by using that grace, each of us will be able to stay faithful to Love.

~⋇~

Today I realized I must have PMDD. The past week has been like a trip to hell and back. I am not totally out yet, but seeing the light. My husband-to-be is sleeping, and I am filled with emotional pain and fear....but I believe that's the PMDD. The extreme negativity was so

powerful this month. I am so grateful that I am more than willing to face this, because I KNOW I act mean to him, and to my sweet mom. The two people I love the most, and my inner self-loathing decides to call some shots. I am aghast at this. I am a little overwhelmed, and, like I said, hurting pretty badly. My significant other really needs his rest, and without this [blog] to focus on I might have woken him crying and begging for his attention. This is a really scary thing. But I know I will find ways to help it and to cope. Thank you for being here, and thank you for listening. Good luck to all the fellows out there who try to understand and offer love during a confusing, painful time.

~ᵥᵢₑ~

First off i want to thank you for this site, it's a great thing you are doing here. Until you, all i ever seemed to find on PMS or PMDD was a simple warning of mood swings and irrational behavior, but no particulars to compare to. What to expect, what's not acceptable.

~ᵥᵢₑ~

In putting in all of this energy to insure she is okay, when do the man's feelings come into it? I noticed through reading your tips for men that it doesn't say a lot about how a man is feeling or could feel in this. I'm not sure if I am the only one who gets Sexually Frustrated out there but when your partner never wants to be intimate due to PMDD & never wants to be intimate when not having an episode either I'm left feeling un-loved, alone,

depressed, sad & more. Is this normal? What do I do to help myself in this situation?

⚜

I'm afraid I can't address how a man is feeling or could feel in this situation since I am not one and I try not to talk about things I don't know about. My goal here is to help women with PMDD to understand what is happening to them in a way they can hopefully share with their partner. My best guess is your situation goes beyond PMDD and therefore I am unable to address it. Because my information shows that a woman with PMDD craves more affection during an episode, but is also super-sensitive to rejection at that time, so if she is not in a positive, healthy, and supportive relationship with someone who understands what is going on, all kinds of things can go wrong.

Each partner has to do their part when it comes to PMDD. If she is not doing hers, then no matter what you do, how understanding and supportive you are, you can't make the relationship work. A good forum for questions like yours can be found at mdjunction.com. Type in the words "PMDD and men" for a list of appropriate forums. The Experience Project also has several pages devoted to sharing stories about PMDD for both men and women. These are personal account sites, not medical information or treatment option sites. Still, you may find some solace in sharing your story with those who understand what you are going through.

⚜

This is such a debilitating, isolating and exhausting condition that I don't even know where to start.

⚜

I'm a stubborn man but not without compassion. I'm 46

and my now ex girl friend is 45.We managed to make it for just over a year. At the beginning it was magical; she would be my last and forever love. She did warn me that she would get severe PMS and that that full moon would also affect her. The episodes would come with no warning, we would have a wonderful evening together and the next morning she would phone me, a totally different person, then the texts would start. At first i would reply but eventually i would put my phone down and walk away. She would attack me on all fronts, my ability as a boyfriend, my ability as a father, where i live, how i live, she would demean the things i'd do for her, and tell me that most everything i bought for her was worthless and ugly, all the way down to my performance in the bedroom. It always starts with her accusing me of cheating.

～⁂～

I am almost positive I suffer from PMDD but have become much more aware of the symptoms in the last few months, I think having the coil fitted could be contributing to this. I am in a new relationship and the last thing I want is for this to be affected by my symptoms. I definitely suffer from the insecurity and paranoia as well as all the rest and I don't know how to raise it with my boyfriend as I don't want him to think I'm mad or that this is a massive problem that is not worth dealing with. Outside of my PMDD I am a very rational and secure person.

～⁂～

After reading the comments above PMDD just seems such a

burden to inflict on someone you love, and particularly someone that is a really good person and just doesn't deserve any of this.

~⋆~

To you husbands and boyfriends...how do we redeem ourselves?? We can't go back and change what we did or said, the guilt stays and the anxiety of knowing that no matter how hard you try, you are going to blow it again... that in itself adds to the stress which in turn worsens our PMDD. How do we reconcile a relationship that we destroy every month??? Is separation the only answer?? Or do we all just suffer on???

~⋆~

I am desperate to find a way to manage this condition before I do any damage to my relationship. It feels like a ticking time bomb and one that I have had to fight tooth and nail to control so far.

~⋆~

This, in essence, is the fundamental struggle between the woman with PMDD and her reptilian PMDD brain. The fight is debilitating, exhausting, and seems endless. Many give up trying. Many medicate to achieve numbness. Fifteen percent of us succeed at killing ourselves. Countless more attempt suicide during our monthly PMDD episodes. PMDD truly is hell on earth for everyone involved.

~⋆~

I love this woman more than she will ever know. I wish i could be stronger for her but her words and actions are destroying what self esteem and confidence i have left.

~⋆~

My other half of 2+ years has PMDD. I have learned to overlook her mood swings and the things she says to me... i know it's not her true real feelings at all. With her i can tell by her tone of voice, and how she types her texts. i guess you can say i read her well. i know it's not good to point out her moods but sometimes it is better to be honest with her. i know throughout this time of the month life can and will be hell. but at the end of the day she is the love of my life and she knows i will walk the fires of hell for her even if they are in our home...

As a man, I am experiencing some extreme frustration dealing with and understanding the unbelievable mood swings presented to me monthly by my girlfriend. I have no other explanation but PMDD. She is in absolute denial about anything being wrong at all. She wants me to apologize for things I do not do or for things that are routine and normal except for during the PMDD time of the month. She is so intelligent and it is hard for me to understand why she does not realize that something is going on.

Ok, I am a wife of a wonderful and loving man who has put up with what I now know is PMDD for 10 years. He feels like he has to goad me all the way to a emotional blowup that includes horrible words and accusations and talk of divorce on both our parts, until I "snap back" and realize I have lost it, which I usually do. Afterward I feel guilty, depressed, and full of shame that I said those horrible things and threw things and have actually slapped him! I don't even know where my hand came from, all of a sudden it was slapping him!?! I am "normally" a kind, happy, loving gal. I fear now that the only resort is to separate and spare us both any more agony.

~·~

I'm writing this when I'm well and happy but the days are ticking down to the full moon (oh yes, in one of life's ironies I not only get PMDD but it hits on the bullseye every full moon). I've lost relationships and many friendships to it. I have become so desperate I'm going to my Ob/Gyn to discuss removal of my remaining ovary (my other ovary was removed due to endometriosis). However I have discovered taking away my right ovary could cause many other serious health issues (turns out the hormones don't just send us loopy, they also perform many other tasks around the body, ie: keeping the heart and brain healthy) so it just may not be viable. So I'm back to thinking about regular exercise, changing my diet drastically for the better etc etc. PMDD is like living with an unstable volcano inside...you never quite know when it's gonna blow...

~·~

I have posted on several different websites about my experiences with dating a girl with PMDD. I spent 3 1/2 years of my life trying to calm my then girlfriend down and to try to get her to seek help. She has a history of problems in her life and also mental illness in her family. I believe that ALL of these problems come from PMDD. Her mother had severe problems and her father couldn't cope with the constant roller coaster ride. He had mental breakdowns and developed an alcohol problem to cope with it. My ex has inherited the wild PMDD mood swings for 2 weeks of EVERY month from her mother. I loved her to bits but my life will be better without her in the long run. The only thing you can do is put up with living on an emotional roller coaster or walk away from a PMDD woman. Sorry, but I tried harder than I have tried at anything in my life and it still didn't work. You would not believe the things she'd say to me/problems she caused. If I had married her it would have ended in divorce as she was so out of control and unstable. Maybe yours isn't as bad but I wish you luck. You may need it...

❧

The best advice I can give is to acknowledge how she feels and put her worries to rest when she isn't voicing them. My girlfriend is so thankful to see that I understand her and I feel like we really make progress. Women with PMDD already feel crazy when they are overwhelmed with these symptoms, so it helps them to relax when they know you understand.

❧

The first step is making the choice to figure it out for the both of you. Then figuring her out, and then you have to figure yourself out, and stop yourself from reacting. Once you've managed all that then you need to try and talk to her, help her help herself. This is hard because as far as she knows, it's you that has the problem.

❧

I am currently having a tough time with these issues, as my girlfriend honestly believes that I provoke her into fights and force her to make amends before the fight will end. I want to accuse her of playing mind games with me because I am often the one to put out the fires after she has a panic attack. It is the hardest thing to be a gentleman and show compassion toward that special woman in your life when she labels you as a horrible person.

~·~

The best treatment that I have found is a non-generic Fluoxetine, Agnus castus, Evening Primrose Oil, B6, D3, Calcium, Zinc, Magnesium, Vitamin C, a healthy diet, very little alcohol, adequate rest, moderate exercise and do not go hungry or starve yourself.

This is what my partner takes and it has returned her back to her normal self. If she misses one part of the above treatment, I know that she will turn into a monster at some point and make my life a living hell.

I hope this information helps someone out there. Female partners in same sex relationships also need advice. I was one of them and I researched the condition and found my girlfriend a really good doctor. Another thing is to be careful when using hormones or the pill to treat PMDD as it can often make it worse.

~·~

I can vouch for all of these: B6, D3, Calcium, Zinc, Magnesium, Vitamin C, a healthy diet, very little alcohol, adequate rest, moderate

136

exercise, and do not go hungry or starve yourself. I don't take the fluoxetine, have never tried Agnus castus, and I took evening primrose years ago but now I take EFAs, or essential fatty acids.

All of the supplements named above I take DAILY, not just in the second two weeks of my cycle. Just be sure to take the B6 along with a quality B50 complex, as the B6 works best in concert with the other B vitamins. Thank you for sharing your "formula" for success!

You are also absolutely right in that using synthetic hormones or contraceptives to treat PMDD can often make your symptoms worse. Each brand of The Pill has a different level of synthetic progesterone (also known as a progestin) in it, and several studies have shown this progestin component of the formula to be the reason moods worsen while on it. Several studies have also shown the estrogen component of birth control pills to increase your chances of suffering from a blood clot, stroke, and/or breast cancer.

How sad is it that so many women would rather risk death than suffer through another episode of PMDD?

~∿~

My partner takes all of this daily. This week she missed a meal and hasn't been taking some of her vitamins. She has been pure hell this week. I want this to end but I love her. It is just so much work and I can't stand the verbal abuse. I wish she would be responsible and just take the medication and supplements and buy more or tell me when they run out! I am so depressed and anxious when she gets like this that I have been considering suicide.

~∿~

I am now giving up. I can't take her abuse anymore. Our relationship was so great to begin with. Now I am frightened and treading on eggshells in our home. She is a monster. Why won't she just take responsibility for her health and even her life? I am ending our 5 year relationship with a sad but relieved heart.

᠁

I diagnosed myself with PMDD a long time ago. I don't want my spouse to feel like some of you—actually I know how it feels because I, too, had a parent with it. It is absolutely miserable to lose your shit every month, to go from confident & fun to irrational & insecure—no way to live.

Chapter Fifteen

————◆————

When Your Partner Won't Get Help

PMDD Wars: Supportive Partners, Women in Denial

Three years after I started my blog in 2010 I learned of a segment of the PMDD population I'd left unaddressed—mainly because I had no idea it existed. My blog posts with tips for men were written in response to the many posts I was seeing from women with unsupportive partners. What, they wanted to know, could they do to help their partners understand their PMDD?

But since 2013 I have heard from both men and women who love their wives and girlfriends, and would be more than willing to do whatever it took to help her to deal with her PMDD....

Only she's not interested. Because she's not the one with the problem, *he* is, and if he can't deal with that, well, then...

Sound familiar?

It happens in a lot of relationships, and not just those involving PMDD. One partner is trying to work things out, and the other is in denial. Unfortunately, this is a sure-fire recipe for failure. For a relationship to succeed it has to have two consenting adults. Two people behaving like grownups, each taking responsibility for their part in making the relationship work—or not work. It's not about power, control, or changing the other person. It's about doing your part to show your partner that your relationship is a priority in your life, and that you want it to last.

You don't do that by:

Playing the blame game

Expecting your partner to change

Trying to change your partner (for their own good or any other reason)

Running from the problem by working too much or never being home

Ignoring your partner's needs

Being abusive to your partner

Denying there is a problem

Relationships require compromise, day in and day out. They're not about one partner giving up all sense of self to cater to the wants and whims of the other. It's a balancing act, and one that needs adjusting and readjusting daily. It's hard enough to have a successful relationship between two healthy people. Throw in some PMDD and your troubles increase exponentially.

But they don't have to. Whether you believe it or not, you **do** have choices when it comes to your PMDD. You can't control when it hits, but you can manage your reaction to it. You can either take the path of least resistance and give in to your seemingly uncontrollable urges, or you can take a stand and say, "I am not my PMDD. I am better than this."

Your PMDD is not who you are, not the real you. Root yourself in this knowledge and stand firm. Refuse to let your PMDD brain get the better of you. Refuse to let the negativity win. Sure, you'll still be weepy and edgy and anxious and irrational at times. Accept that that happens, but don't let it have free rein during an episode. We all slip up now and then, but to totally immerse yourself in the negativity and irrationality...that doesn't do anybody any good—yourself, your partner, or your children.

Think of your children if you can't think of anything else. Don't they deserve better than to see you not even *trying* to get along with your chosen mate?

This completely boggles my mind. I myself entered a PMDD episode recently. I knew it was coming, I could feel the storm approaching, and all I wanted to do was to be held. Unfortunately, the circumstances for that to happen didn't fall in line. It was payday and my husband was feeling flush. He called and asked if I wanted to go out to dinner at our favorite restaurant.

I reluctantly said sure. I was only going to heat up leftovers anyway. Now I wouldn't have to do even that. In short, I adapted. I decided to let myself be pampered another way since I couldn't have what I really wanted.

But all night long, he kept asking, "Is something wrong? You seem distracted."

Something was wrong, and I *was* distracted, but distraction is also an occupational hazard for a writer, so he's used to it.

Finally I said, "I can feel the storm coming."

He knew what I meant.

He took me home and I went right to bed.

We spent the day apart on Saturday, seeing to individual tasks. I felt all right most of the day, probably because I didn't have to interact with anyone, but around 5:00 p.m. I had an intense craving for carbs.

I ate a bowl of cereal with almond milk. Shortly thereafter my husband arrived and off we went to church...where I could not stay focused to save myself. My mind bounced from thought to thought to thought.

Afterward, now out of almond milk, we went to the grocery store. I had three things I wanted to get: almond milk, Brazil nuts (for selenium), and cat food. It took every ounce of my concentration to stay on task, to simply remember those three items, and remember where each was located in the store. Since by now I was feeling completely miserable—head pounding, joints aching, brain feeling like it was on fire—my mission was to get in, get my stuff, and get out.

In church, I had let my mind wander, but now, I had to corral all those bouncing thoughts and force my mind to stay on track. So deliberately focused was I that the minute we arrived in the parking lot, I jumped out of the car and made a beeline for the store, completely ignoring my husband. As soon as I entered the store, I saw the rack where I had last found the Brazil nuts.

In that moment, nothing could have come between me and my goal.

But they were out of Brazil nuts. They had almonds, walnuts, pecans...but no Brazil nuts. My husband caught up with me as I stood in front of the nut rack, feeling completely derailed and wanting to weep.

I turned to him and said, "I want to cry, because there are no Brazil nuts here."

I then asked him, "Am I acting strange?"

And he said, "Yes, I noticed something was off in church."

"I thought so," I said. "It's that time again. I'm having an episode."

I then turned away and went in search of the milk, once again leaving him behind. As I was walking, I realized I was being rude. I then recalled other times I had walked off without him and realized that **each and every time** it was during an episode of PMDD.

Suddenly it hit me that I wasn't **trying** to be rude—it was literally taking every ounce of energy I had to stay on task. Otherwise I might look left or right, get distracted and we'd be wandering the store looking at nothing in particular until my husband said, "Come on, let's go."

I would then burst into tears for no apparent reason, he would wonder what the hell happened, and our evening would be ruined.

I stopped and explained this to him and we finished our shopping together.

But the whole time, I was feeling very angsty and edgy and

primed to have a fight. As he helped me out of the car when we got home, I said to him, "I could start a fight with you so easily right now."

He looked at me in surprise. "About what?"

"That's just it," I said. "About nothing."

I was overtired and achy and weepy and feeling like a toddler on the verge of a tantrum. No lie. Instead I went to bed. Because I know the difference between me and my PMDD.

And because our relationship matters to me.

It might not have been the most exciting ending to the evening, but at least it wasn't filled with a lot of drama that would leave each of us feeling devastated and alone. My husband understood my need for rest and solitude because I was able to express it in a quiet and (somewhat) rational matter. My husband understands my sudden rudeness and self-absorption is not a reflection of him, but rather of my PMDD.

With a different person, it could have gone completely differently.

If I had behaved differently, it could have gone completely differently.

Because inside of me was someone dying for a fight. It didn't matter what the fight was about. All I wanted to do was goad my husband into sparring with me until I could no longer stand my own irrationality and then burst into the tears I so desperately wanted to weep—and blame him for ruining everything. Maybe even blame him for abandoning me or not loving me when he walked out the door in sheer frustration, for lack of knowing what else to do.

Not because he doesn't love me. But because I wouldn't **let** him love me. Wouldn't let him see my need, my vulnerability, my (what my reptilian PMDD brain would call) weakness, and wouldn't **trust** him to take care of me.

Think about it: Which would you rather be...lovingly cared for, or crying and alone?

I'm still having an episode. My head still pounds, my eyes hurt, my joints hurt, my back hurts, my brain burns, and I want to cry. There is no doubt I could be drawn into an argument, any argument, with anyone, at the drop of a hat. It may still happen...because sometimes the strength to hold the negativity at bay just isn't there.

But I do know that if it happens, it will only be for a moment, before I catch myself again, and remind myself that I am not my PMDD, and that my blindsided target doesn't deserve to be abused just because I am having a bad day.

No one does.

~~~

PMDD and Denial

So what did I do two weeks ago when I was hit with my latest double header? (Sometimes the PMDD comes *twice* a month, lucky me, and sometimes not at all, due to my increasing age and anovulatory (no egg released) cycles. If no egg is released, you don't get PMDD.)

So yes, this means that this past month, I experienced two PMDD episodes—right on schedule. The first one was to, um, celebrate ovulation, and the second was for the really Big Show...also known as Waiting for Red.

Anyway, while I was in the PMDD zone, I worked, I

wrote, and I slept. (Three hour naps are not unusual when my hormonal system gets so far out of whack.) I focused on survival only. I pared my life down to the bare bones, ate take-out from the organic co-op or heated up all-natural frozen entrees, focused on my work (I work at home, due in part to my PMDD), and wrote my heart out. I took walks when I needed a boost in my feel good hormones. Took time out for me.

But I didn't do any of that until I finally admitted I was having a problem. And so, it got me to thinking. Why was it I waited so long to admit my PMDD was acting up again? Why was I so deep in denial?

Because I had work to do, a schedule to maintain, a life to live. I didn't have time to give in to some strange, intangible brain disorder that keeps me from getting the things done I want and need to get done.

I wanted to be normal.

I cannot emphasize enough how much women with PMDD want to feel normal. We don't want to admit there's something going on in our brains that isn't right. Something that even the medical professionals can't agree on, much less define. We can find a thousand excuses for why we are so clumsy at times, or so ravenous, or irritable, edgy, disoriented, anxious, or weepy. We deny and deny and deny there is anything wrong with us, or that we are in any way acting strangely, because to admit that we are doing so means we will have to stop and deal with it somehow, and how can you deal with something that defies description?

Sometimes it's a battle you just don't want to fight.

Somehow we've convinced ourselves it's easier to ignore the

symptoms we can't explain and plow onward. Because that's what women do. We keep going until we can't go any more. Women with PMDD are especially strong and stubborn in this regard. We go and go and go until we collapse. Or until our behavior becomes so erratic that someone in our life can't stand it anymore and says, "What's *wrong* with you?"

Even then we deny it. There's nothing wrong with me. If you'd just pick up your clothes, fix the faucet, turn down the TV, do your homework, call me, stop calling me, show up on time, take the trash out, *talk* to your parent/child/boss/sibling, move your car, paint the bedroom, fill out the report, mail the letter, do what I ask, everything would be fine. The problem is you, not me. *You're* what's wrong with me.

And off we head into another relationship disaster, be it with our children, parents, co-workers, siblings or partners.

The bottom line is there *is* something wrong with us. But it's not something we have any control over, any more than we have control over our genetic predisposition to any number of diseases, eye color, or shoe size. And it's not something we can explain, unless we've done a whole boatload of research—only to find out it's different for every woman, because we each live in different circumstances and environments and the biological rhythms of our bodies are unique to each of us. No two women are alike. Some have some symptoms, others have others. They come at different times of the month. Before periods, after periods, some even before and/or after ovulation. Sometimes it's two short episodes, sometimes the episode starts with ovulation and stays with the woman all the way through menstruation. It can get as bad as leaving the woman with only ONE good week per month.

Who wants to live like that?

My point is we don't have control over when or how often it happens, or how long it chooses to stay, but we *do* have control over how we respond to our PMDD.

And denial is just not an option. Not if you don't want to leave a landscape littered with big mistakes, bad decisions, and tattered and broken relationships behind you everywhere you go.

To get a handle on your PMDD, you need to get a handle on yourself. You need to find a way to spend time on you, spend some time with yourself, getting to know your body and your unique hormonal rhythms. You need peace and quiet to do this. You can't do this in the middle of your latest financial, household, work, school, or family crisis. You also need to like yourself to do this. You need to believe you are worth the time and effort.

Sometimes I feel like I live a totally self-indulgent life. I do what I want to do, go where I want to go, see who I want to see, and generally manage my life so that it encounters the least amount of stress and conflict. No drama queen here. I don't have time for drama. It only sets off my PMDD, and God knows I don't want any more experiences with that if I can help it.

So I take care of myself. I eat right, I exercise, I manage my stress. And even then I still get hit with the occasional strong episode of PMDD.

But just imagine if I didn't do all of that. How out of control my life would be. How joyless, how miserable, how sad and self-destructive.

Ignoring your PMDD is like ignoring a train bearing down on you. A wreck is inevitable. Studies have shown that if you leave your PMDD untreated, it will only grow worse over time, and you have a very good chance of ending up with Major Depressive Disorder. Is this what you want for your life? I know it's not what I want. I also know that ignoring my PMDD, denying it, doesn't make me more normal at all.

It only makes things worse.

There are, however, many things you can do to lessen the severity of your symptoms, and most of those things are mentioned either in this book, or somewhere on my blog, and are also free, or relatively inexpensive.

Which is why you don't hear a lot about them. The only ones you hear about are the ones people are making money off of. But no magic pill is going to cure your PMDD, no matter how much you hope it will. PMDD is not a one-size-fits-all disorder. We've got to stop treating it like it is. Putting women with PMDD on oral contraceptives or antidepressants to suppress (not solve) their hormonal issues is like asking every woman to wear a tent dress. It might cover the body, but it's not a good fit.

It's also a huge form of denial. Denial of our individuality, and denial of our biology.

So the first step is to **stop denying we have a problem**. Forty years later, I'm still guilty of doing it, even with all that I have learned about the disorder. Is it any wonder those who haven't done the research I have are equally caught up in denial? And what about the women who don't know PMDD exists? All they do is run around thinking they're crazy, desperate to deny it to themselves and everyone else.

You can't possibly think that to wake up one morning feeling fine, then slowly start to lose your fine motor skills, become agitated and confused, weepy, exhausted, irritable, and ravenous before dinner time is normal. The ability to wash away all of that with 45 minutes of aerobic exercise is also not normal. The fact that doing so buys you a couple of hours of PMDD-free time is not normal. The inevitable drop in mood and energy level when it wears off is also not normal.

But it is what it is, and it's all we've got to work with. PMDD doesn't do normal. Accept that and just do what you can to get through it. Surround yourself with people who will support you in your efforts toward good health and wellness. Weed out the people in your life that don't. Take time for yourself, be good to yourself, and most of all, when the episodes come…don't deny them. Just find your own way to relax and go with the flow—no pun intended.

Chapter Sixteen

Some Final Comments From Readers

Random comments from readers: *Responses from me are in italics.*

$\sim\!\!\checkmark\!\!\sim$

My wife and I have been together for 17 years and I've only just discovered your blog. For 17 years I've wondered exactly what has been wrong, and now I finally know, just at the moment when I really honestly don't know if I can continue to take the roller-coaster that PMDD puts you on. It's totally devastating to a stable marriage to have one spouse demonstrate how much she loves you and her life for part of every month, and then demonstrate how much she loathes you (and perhaps even the children) the other part. It's like living with Jekyll & Hyde.

$\sim\!\!\checkmark\!\!\sim$

My wife is expert at hiding her PMDD from everyone else. Only our children and I understand what happens to her. She holds it in around everyone else, but then at home we bear the brunt of her pent up frustrations, which is just the PMDD talking. But it hurts all of us badly nonetheless.

~*/~

Exactly the same for me, but for even longer. My wife refuses to even recognize that there's a problem. In some ways, that is the most destructive part. I can't begin to say how devastating it has been. I am simply exhausted. Jekyll and Hyde doesn't come close. You give so much love and get slaughtered in return.

~*/~

About seeking treatment, or refusing to, that's part of the PMDD. When things are going well, we feel normal, and see no need to seek treatment, because everything is fine, thank you, and when we are having a PMDD episode, we're trying so hard to ignore it and simply function, that we're either deep in denial, or too depressed to do anything about it. Then, of course, the PMDD brain takes over and treatment is not an option. Also, many women have tried to seek help and been met with ignorance and/or disbelief because their doctors either don't understand PMDD or don't have the time or inclination to learn more about it. It's easier just to prescribe antidepressants and move on to the next patient.

It's hard to be your own best advocate when you're going through these bewildering cycles of anger, depression, anxiety, and feeling somewhat normal. You never know who you're going to be from day to day. Also, when you make an appointment, you're usually at the point where you can't stand it anymore and desperately want help, but then the appointment is three weeks away and by that time, all your symptoms are gone…until the next time. If you're in the middle of an episode when you have your appointment, it's hard to clearly explain what is happening, because your brain simply isn't working right. You can't get the words out, and instead you end up losing it, breaking down in tears, then go home feeling like more of a failure than when you left for the appointment.

So…It's hard to convince a doctor you have a problem when you seem perfectly fine, and your doctor is more likely to think you need mental health counseling if you show up angry, anxious, depressed, and crying. Either way, women with PMDD lose when reaching out for help to doctors unfamiliar with PMDD.

~✵~

We did have a three month break earlier this year. But then we got back together. Everything was fantastic! We were talking about living together and how we might plan our wedding. Then she became distant again. When I brought up the idea that she may have PMDD, she said she was fine for the three months we had been apart. She did date someone briefly in that time. Is it possible her PMDD could be less severe and more like PMS symptoms for that three months because she was kind of in escape mode…not dating anyone seriously? When we did get back together, she told me he was nothing…just a distraction. What are your thoughts?

~✵~

It's possible she was fine for the three months she was away. Put it this way: If she was seeing someone else he was new and a mystery and at that point things are usually pretty rosy and you are looking at things you have in common, things to bring you closer (this is whether it be with a love interest or even just a friend to hang out with), vs things to move you apart. All this finding common ground increases the level of your bonding hormones and in my experience, oxytocin trumps PMDD every time. Nothing like a good surge of oxytocin (in my case cuddling with my husband) to make the PMDD blues go away.

This is not to say she was cuddling with anyone…simply the fantasy of cuddling with someone (even a movie star) can generate the same biological results in your brain. Talking to a friend and feeling heard or understood can generate the same biological feelings; as can cuddling with a baby or playing with a puppy or kitten. Oxytocin makes no distinction between whether it's a pet or a person, or even just being good to yourself. That's why I encourage women with PMDD to take time out and be good to themselves during an episode of PMDD. Rest, relax, do whatever boosts your oxytocin levels and makes you feel ready to face the world again.

So…If she was in escape mode and determined to believe that all was well in her world, then it is quite possible her brain chemistry reflected that feeling and the PMDD was held at bay during those months. Most couples who are genuinely interested in each other have their first major argument within three months… (if one party is not genuinely interested in having a relationship it can and usually does come much sooner), but at that point a healthy couple decides if they want to split or keep trying…and continues to do so with every major disagreement.

If she truly doesn't see the relationship working out, then there is nothing you can do about it, but quite often that is the PMDD talking.

You can't see the positive in anything when you're having an episode of PMDD, and the PMDD brain magnifies the negative at least tenfold.

She would have to cooperate with you to learn to manage her PMDD—and you'd both have to refrain from making major decisions of any sort during PMDD episodes—or your life on this emotional roller coaster will only get worse.

So while I applaud your decision to stand by your PMDD woman, just remember you can't fix something YOU didn't break. Since it affects both of you, it takes both of you to get a handle on her PMDD.

⸲⸲⸲

I'm new to this PMDD thing... but I have read at TON on it. I think you are right... There just may be something else going on here than just her PMDD. Her direct, deep cutting insults and criticisms go above and beyond in my opinion. My suggestion is to get out and get your sanity back. Take care of yourself. Hang out with friends of similar mind set. Do some work on YOU! And READ everything you can about PMDD.

Chapter Seventeen

———— ◆ ————

Inside the Mind of a Woman with PMDD

The Other Side of PMDD

My wife has PMDD 2 weeks each month. I can now track it on a calendar. The meanness, sharp tongue, irritability, over-sensitivity to the slightest comment... it's all there each month, like clockwork. I used to make the mistake of reacting to her negativity, which results in a showdown at the OK Corral with talks of divorce, etc., etc. Now, I just keep my mouth shut, offer my help, not reacting to the negativity. It's not easy at all. My only escape is to go to the gym when it seems everything I do is wrong in her eyes. But I bear it each month because I love my wife and I know it's not her. I say she becomes Mr. Hyde once a month for 2 weeks, and I just learn to keep my mouth shut. A big exercise in tolerance and patience. If you love your wife or special someone, tolerance and patience are vital. If you don't have them, you will suffer.

⁓ᵛ⁄ᵉ⁓

This man is suffering. My heart goes out to him. My admiration and respect go out to him as well, because he loves his wife and refuses to let her PMDD ruin, end, or dissolve their marriage.

What he says is true. "If you love your wife or special someone, tolerance and patience are vital. If you don't have them, you will suffer."

I suspect he is talking about himself, here, but he could just as easily be talking about both of them.

Much is made over the suffering of the non-PMDD partner in a relationship. But let me say this—as much as you are suffering by being the brunt of her emotions, she is suffering at least twice as much on the inside. She doesn't want to be doing what she is doing. She is often as horrified as you are by what comes out of her mouth. Yes, in that moment a part of her malfunctioning brain wants you to suffer as she is suffering, but overall, none of us *wants* to have PMDD, much less *every month*.

Let's do the math. The average age of female puberty is 12; the average age of menopause is 51. Round that off to 40 years of menstruation. Multiply that by 12; that gives you 480 months of periods if you never have children, less if you do. Let's go with 450 periods for now. That gives you 900 weeks of pre-menstrual issues. Divide that by 52 weeks per year, and you get 17+ years that a woman can spend in the living hell that is PMDD.

157

Seventeen *years,* people!

So yes, to partners like the man on the previous page, I am grateful beyond measure. One, because you treat your wife with love and respect, and two, because you have allowed me to see where you are coming from, and to respond to what you see from the outside with what is happening to me on the inside.

Notice I didn't say what is happening to *your* loved one with PMDD. That, I cannot know for sure, but by explaining what happens to me, I might be able to open the door to a conversation between the two of you about what happens to her.

I'm going through an episode right now. It started about two days ago. I'd like to say I can pinpoint when the slide began, but I cannot. It seems like a gradual shift, a slow sinking into the darkness—as opposed to coming out of an episode, which I have literally felt in my head when my "non-PMDD brain" snapped back into place. The return to sanity can be instantaneous. The gradual slide into anger, despair, and hopelessness can take what feels like forever.

So while this is what you are seeing on the outside—a moody, irrational, unreasonable, emotional, maybe rude, unfocused, uncaring, disoriented, scattered or otherwise strangely acting woman—I'm going to tell you what's happening on the inside. My head hurts, my bones hurt, my joints and muscles hurt. I didn't want to wake up this morning. I feel like I have been drugged. My mouth is dry and there is a tightness behind my eyes reminiscent of a hangover, but I have not had any alcohol. I feel fat and smelly and ugly.

Yesterday, in the hopes of cheering myself up, I decided to

organize the photos from a trip to Alaska with friends. In every single photo I was in, I hated how I looked. Normally, my looks do not bother me. I know I am me, and I am loved just the way I am. Yesterday, I was obsessed with my body image. Couldn't find enough flaws to point out to myself.

Okay, so that project didn't turn out. Yesterday, I also went to a funeral. It might not have been the best of ideas, but really, you have no choice when these things happen. You either go or you don't. I felt paying my respects was more important than hiding in my cave. I waited until the last half hour of the viewing, so that if anything went awry, I had a natural exit. As it turned out, there were several people there I would have loved to have talked with longer. Sad circumstances, but I enjoyed seeing them all again just the same.

The funeral itself was lovely and poignant...one of the most beautiful services I have attended...

But it sparked thoughts of death and dying for the rest of the day. Who's going to go next? How long do I have? How many of us will be here next year? What do I want to do with the time I have left?

This very question nearly devolved into an argument between me and my husband last night. Normally I am happy to live in the moment and let life unfold as it will. Last night there was an urgency, an almost desperation behind my thoughts and words. We need to do this, and we need to do that, and we need to do it NOW.

I will feel very foolish when that feeling goes away in a week. I know this already.

If he had argued with me instead of patiently "listened" to

me I would have (at least mentally) declared the relationship hopeless and over. There would have been harsh words and an explosion of tears. I suppose I should be happy that I'm only going to feel foolish. Especially if he takes my dark words to heart...while I've blissfully gone back to my "It's all good" mode.

If you were my husband, wouldn't you be confused?

Another example: Our church music minister plays guitar, has a beautiful voice, and chooses upbeat songs. Normally I love to sing along with her. Last night her music irritated the hell out of me. Like fingernails on a chalkboard. She didn't do anything different. *I* was the one who was different.

Inside. Inside I was different. But I never let on, not on the outside. If I had, I'd only come off as crazy.

When we got back to the car, after a very uplifting service, I told my husband, "Right now, I could tell you what is wrong with anything. You just name it, and I will tell you what is wrong with it."

This is where the "I can't do anything right" mentality comes from in partners of women with PMDD.

I spent most of yesterday alone, as my husband was busy elsewhere. (He has learned when to leave me alone.) Even while my PMDD self was irritated beyond words at supposedly "being abandoned" I was glad he was not here, having to bear the brunt of my irrationality. I knew, as he would have known had he been here, that there was absolutely nothing he could do right yesterday.

So it was best that he was elsewhere. The same went for my son. He walked in the door, aiming for a quick change of clothes, and within two minutes I was not speaking to him. It was best for him, and for me. He left after giving me a big hug and telling me he loves me. As I shut the door behind him my thoughts were, "Yeah, right."

I adore my son, and we get along great. Anybody who knows us knows he loves me, too. He can get manipulative, like kids do, and I let him, like Moms do, but the love is always there.

Not yesterday. Even though it was being freely offered, I wasn't feeling it.

Yesterday I was feeling my most unlovable. Old, dumb, lazy, overwhelmed, uncertain, weepy, morbid, incompetent, uncaring, and unkind. In real life, I am none of those things. If anyone had been around me yesterday...if I had not spent the day alone (except for the funeral)...I would have snapped and snarled all day.

Why?

Because I was feeling extremely vulnerable. I was feeling worthless, useless, and like every decision I'd ever made in my life was wrong.

Hello?

For one, that's not even possible. But there you go.

PMDD doesn't make sense.

So you're walking around feeling gross physically, mentally, and emotionally, and you just...well, you're miserable inside. Nothing can make you happy, and nobody better try, because if they try they will fail— you'll see to that—and if they don't try, well, you'll have something to say about that, too.

It's no wonder I get letters from women with PMDD who

fear they will spend the rest of their lives alone. Who can deal with someone like that? Where nothing you do is right for days, sometimes weeks, on end.

Yesterday I could have gone on a rant like you wouldn't believe about what was wrong in my life.

Funny, I was perfectly happy with my life three days ago. Feeling rather blessed, actually.

This personality change is bewildering enough to watch from the outside. Try to imagine what it feels like from the inside. Try to imagine your brain feeding you lies *all day long*. Nobody likes you, everybody hates you, you're nothing but a big screw-up, a slob, a loser, a bad (mom, sister, daughter, friend, wife, girlfriend—fill in the blank). You're dumb and disorganized, lazy and useless, your life is a mess, and even your own (dog, cat, turtle, fill in the blank here) hates you....

You spend all your energy either fighting off these lies in your head, or letting them wear you down, beat you down. Like I said—and I got this from a blog post I read years ago—PMDD is a bully. So here you are, being bullied by your PMDD brain. You're feeling your worst, and your weakest—your most vulnerable. Your PMDD has come around to kick you while you are down, for the PMDD brain shows no mercy.

Someone says something to you. In your PMDD state, your brain twists that something around to the most negative interpretation possible.

What are you going to do...fight or flight?

The primitive brain (aka my PMDD brain) has me fighting. That's where my brain goes during PMDD. Into primitive, reptilian, survival mode. It's fight or flight, survival of the fittest, baby, and I'm going to see to it that you go down in flames, no matter what the cost to our relationship.

The opposite of fighting is withdrawal. Withdrawal into ourselves—where we let the PMDD bully run rampant inside us—and withdrawal into depression—where we accept what the PMDD bully says, and beat ourselves up even after he or she is long gone.

Try living with a bully inside your brain for two weeks a month and see how long *you* last before you lose it one way or another. Either through anger or tears, or both. So yes, while it is undoubtedly hard on our partners and the friends and family who love us, keep in mind that PMDD is no picnic for the woman herself. She is doing the best she can with a temporarily malfunctioning brain. The woman you love is having technical difficulties. Her brain is literally not firing on all cylinders. She doesn't *want* to ruin your party, your weekend, your vacation, relationship, or marriage.

She just wants to feel safe, from demons neither of you can understand nor see.

~

The Other Side of PMDD, continued

Since I wrote that last section, and since I was PMDD-ing this week, I paid close attention to what was going on inside my head. Thursday I was overwhelmed and angry. Normally I love to feed people, take care of them, give them a hot meal and some home comforts. But my husband, son, and I had agreed it would be "fend for yourself" night on Thursdays, due to different commitments. I was therefore "supposed" to worry only about myself.

But then they both showed up at dinnertime, hungry and neither one of them cooks. So instead of just worrying about myself, I was suddenly in charge of a meal, and in no mood to graciously pull one together. Instead I became like a drill sergeant...you, go and set the table...you, chop those vegetables...you're in charge of the microwave...you, get us something to drink.

Not my usual self at all, but I rose to the occasion and kept a lid on my resentments. Even so, later on in the evening, after we'd come and gone to the Christmas show we were all trying to get to on time, I apologized to my husband for being so...well...bossy.

He didn't mind. He said, "You hardly ever get like that. It's nice to see you're human."

This got me to really thinking about PMDD and what's going on inside our heads when it happens. Are we really screwing up, or is our PMDD brain telling us we're screwing up when we are not, and that's what fuels our insecurities and ignites our fights and relationship issues?

Because you know when you're screwing up. Everyone does, except the truly mentally ill. But those of us who aren't don't need people to tell us when we mess up. Because we know it, inside, when we make a genuine mistake. Pointing our failures out to us only makes things worse. (And I am talking about human beings here, not just women with PMDD.) Men and women alike, we all get hurt and defensive and either go into withdrawal or denial—or come out fighting.

So here's my thought: What if we're not really screwing

up—our PMDD brain has simply convinced us that we are, and so we act accordingly—by coming out fighting? Science tells us that during an episode of PMDD the fight or flight response kicks in—or, rather, the response kicks in, but then doesn't leave like it's supposed to. Instead, the switch stays on for the entire episode, which, as we all know, can last for weeks. Remember, the brain PET scans of a woman with PMDD are the same as those of a combat veteran with PTSD. During an episode of PMDD, I can say for sure that your loved one definitely feels like she is under fire—from any and all sources.

It's something to consider, the way our PMDD brains deliberately twist our thoughts to create the most negative impact. Because while I thought I was being overly bossy...he just thought I was trying to get everyone fed and out the door in time.

Fast forward to Saturday afternoon. I am in a rage. I know I am in a rage. Thank goodness I am alone. I think that is part of why I am in a rage. I don't want to be alone. I'm tired of working (I work at home), and I want to take a break, do something fun.

But at the same time I know that if someone shows up, my husband or my son, that's not going to make me happy, either. I know this, because in that moment, nothing can make me happy.

So it was best that they each had something else to do for most of the day.

But meanwhile I stewed. And anything and everything that didn't normally bother me suddenly bothered me, big time.

By the time my husband arrived to go to church, I was

angry and I. Just. Didn't. Care.

But I had spent the day "watching" myself, or practicing awareness, so I knew I was angry, and I knew there was no reason (aside from my hormones) for me to be angry, and I knew I was being irrational, and I knew I didn't want a fight.

So I asked him...Do you ever feel like you Just. Don't. Care? You don't care whose feelings you hurt, or who you piss off, or what people think? You've just had it, and you're just going to say and do what you want to say and do?

He said yes, he had felt like that.

I said, "Well, that's the way I feel right now. Like I am going to say and do what I want to, and nobody better get in my way."

"I see," he said.

"I'm just warning you," I said. "I'm in that kind of mood. So that if I do or say something totally irrational, you don't sit there wondering, 'What just happened?'"

"Oh. Okay."

And that was the extent of it. There was no incident. We had no argument. We went to church, and then we rented a movie. We had a perfectly pleasant evening.

But I felt better letting him know what was going on inside of me, so that should I snap, he wasn't taken by surprise.

He appreciated knowing I was on the edge. We settled into a quiet evening together.

"So you can control it?" he asked at one point.

Well...yes, and no.

I can control it up to a point. But when the dam bursts, it bursts. And at that point, I can't control it.

My goal is to keep that dam from bursting. To keep from snapping out on those closest to me.

Because it is my goal, I am getting more and more successful at accomplishing it. But I can tell you of a thousand times where I failed.

Try to imagine walking around with a totally irrational "Don't f*ck with me" attitude going on inside your head. Try to imagine this happening several days a month, like clockwork. It switches on, it shuts off. You have no control over when it does either. All you can do is hang on and hope you (and your relationships) survive the ride.

For instance...take a totally normal exchange at the deli counter when you're in one of these moods.

The deli clerk asks what I would like. I smile and tell her. The clerk asks "sliced or shaved?" This question totally pisses me off inside. I'm here every f*cking week (not true) ordering the same damn thing (close, but also not true) so why can't they f*cking remember (unreasonable expectation) what I like?

Are you seeing how a PMDD mind works?

Meanwhile, I am still smiling and politely answering, "sliced" like I do every time, and feeling like I want to punch the next person who crosses my path.

It's really not about you. (Although it can be, so don't think you're completely off the hook). It's about doing battle with thoughts that come out of nowhere and are sometimes voiced before you can stop them. It's about hearing or seeing or doing something and placing the most negative context on it that you can possibly imagine. It's about not knowing what you want or how to make it better.

167

As I told my husband, "Don't even try to make me feel better right now because you literally can't. You will not be able to win, no matter what you do."

But there are things we can do to keep it from getting worse. Here are some I prefer. Sitting quietly together, watching a movie or maybe listening to music, or taking a nap, or reading a book. Hugging without talking. Going for a walk. Just being together in silence, or at least a peaceful atmosphere.

Figure out what you enjoy or can tolerate. Communicate that to your loved ones.

For me, silence is best, so that I can concentrate on doing battle with the misperceptions raging inside my head. So that I don't suffer information overload and say something I will regret. In short, when I am PMDD-ing, don't confuse me by asking questions, or by wanting something from me. I am using every ounce of control I have to appear sane. This is a time you either need to give to me (your love and understanding) or get the hell out of my way.

There's really no in-between.

PMDD Flashback #3

It's My Party and I'll Cry If I Want To

I got my first inklings something was up on Sunday morning, when I woke up groggy, head hurting, and ravenous. Determined to beat the PMDD blues, I ate a bowl of Cheerios (quick acting carbs) and went back to sleep for another sleep cycle, about an hour and a half. The next time I woke up I felt better, more on an even keel thanks to the carbs and the extra sleep cycle, so I vowed to not let my PMDD ruin "my" day.

And it didn't. Not that day or the next. It was my birthday and almost nothing could get me down, although at the oddest times, I found myself looking off into the distance and just wanting to cry.

That was Sunday. Tuesday I embarked on a project that would challenge anyone's ability to concentrate. For hours I sifted through airline websites and travel reservation matrixes, trying to find the best dates, flight times, and price for two seats to Europe—a gift from my husband. The print function on my computer wouldn't cooperate, so I had to hold all the information in my head from screen to screen to screen. My desk was littered with sticky notes on which I'd scribbled the names of potential destinations, airlines, and prices.

So...flights finally chosen, I'm now filling out the information. Here's something new. I need to input the names of who will be traveling exactly as they appear on the identification we will be using—in this case our passports. I call my husband. He doesn't know what his passport says. He says he will check and call me back in less than an hour.

He gets busy and forgets.

My day takes a nosedive. By the time I see him that evening, I'm not speaking to him.

It's that simple.

I busted my brain on the computer for several hours trying to organize a trip *he* suggested. *He* forgets to make a f*cking 30 second phone call. I am furious. Just that fast. And there is nothing he can do to make it right. And I mean no-thing. I am in the mood for a fight. And I don't care who I fight with. My son makes an equally available target. He disappears into his room as I start sniping at both of them, sharp tones and snide comments left and right. I know I am doing it, and *I don't care.* I feel unloved, unappreciated, unheard, unhappy, unhealthy, unfit, un-everything. You name it. No one understands me. No one cares. No one appreciates the things I do around here.

"I see the weekend is over," my husband says quietly.

We had an amazing weekend. Truly amazing. Went to church, went for a sunset walk, went to a festival, met all sorts of interesting people, played miniature golf, went for a drive in the country, cooked a couple of fantastic dinners, slow danced...he even presented me with a 30 minute DVD of a slide show of my trip to Alaska, set to soothing music. It was my birthday and it was beautiful.

But all of that was gone in my PMDD mind. All that mattered to me right then and there was he didn't call me back; he didn't appreciate my time, my work, or me.

His quiet words were my cue that I had crossed the line.

I apologized. Sincerely. Because I knew I was wrong. In the

end, though, I went to bed and again, just wanted to cry.

The next morning I didn't want to wake up. All morning I couldn't concentrate, couldn't stay focused on any one task. Couldn't even contemplate writing anything. By afternoon, my brain literally hurt, like it was inflamed or something, and I found myself reaching for my PMDD comfort foods...almonds, cheese, chocolate, and oranges.

By evening I knew why.

My period had arrived.

PMDD Flashback #4

The Queen of Denial

She's baaaack! I'm talking about my PMDD self. After several months of relatively mild episodes, suddenly I'm hit with a humdinger. I am one of the unfortunate many who have atypical PMDD, (as I mentioned in my PMDD Flashback #2 - A Perfect Storm of PMDD), in that it occurs both before and after I menstruate. Kind of like a hurricane, with menstruation in the middle, serving as the eye of the storm, where I might feel lousy physically, but I'm clear-headed and things are relatively calm.

So, about ten days ago, I could feel a storm blowing in. I notice I'm starting to get agitated about things that don't usually faze me. I realize I am emotionally looking for a fight, anywhere I can find it. I check the calendar, confirm it's about that time of the month, and warn those closest to me it may be a rocky few days. I back away from conversations and situations I know will set me off, and postpone any important decisions or discussions.

The storm came and went, no major incidents, other than a couple of afternoon naps due to extreme sleepiness. My menses came, and life was good again, aside from the physical discomforts of having a period.

Usually, the second half of my PMDD begins on Day 3 of my period. So when Day 3 came and went with no trouble, I thought I was in the clear, home free, another PMDD episode averted. Kudos to me once again for not letting my PMDD brain get the better of me and wreaking all sorts of havoc in my life and personal relationships.

But this was not my usual period. This one lasted six days instead of three. Not a problem. I'm okay. Life is still good.

But then yesterday morning, I started noticing things. Like I tried to address an envelope, and my handwriting was all jumpy and spiky, like that of an older person. My hand couldn't control the pen the way it usually does. My typing was off, too. I kept hitting the wrong keys.

No matter. I'm just in a hurry. (Denial #1)

Then I went to a funeral at a church I had never been to before. I got lost. Suddenly I'm feeling anxious, edgy, confused, my thoughts all scattered.

No biggie, it can happen to anyone. (Denial #2)

At the funeral, all I wanted to do was weep.

Not a problem. People are supposed to be sad at funerals. (Denial #3)

I came home and fixed myself something to eat. I work at home, so I started to work in my sun-drenched living room. Suddenly I couldn't keep my eyes open any longer.

Nothing unusual there. The room was warm and I had just eaten. Never mind that the room is equally warm and sunny most days, and I eat lunch every day about the same time and don't get sleepy. (Denial #4)

Finally I give in and take a nap, unable to concentrate or stay awake. It still hasn't dawned on me, what is happening, because Day 3 came and went and I escaped the bully's wrath this time around.

I wake up, totally ravenous, and wanting nothing but CHOCOLATE.

Still haven't caught on. Or if I have, I'm heading into serious denial: *I don't have time for this nonsense. It's Day 6 and my PMDD is supposed to be over, dammit! I have work to do.*

A friend calls. We agree to meet up later on, go to our movement and stretching class together. I want to know how soon "later on" is. Is it 4:30, 5:30, 6:30? If it's sooner rather than later, I'll wait to eat with my friend. If it's later, I'll eat now. No big deal either way. I just want to know, so I can plan my evening meal accordingly.

Somehow that simple conversation goes totally awry, and I end up in tears.

Bingo. My evil twin has struck again. Now I know what's going on. My PMDD self has returned for round two. My head hurts, my eyes hurt, all I want to do is cry and go back to sleep. But I'm too agitated and upset to go back to sleep, and I'm so hungry I want to scream. But I just ate a full meal a couple of hours ago. There's no logical reason for me to feel so hungry.

My friend calls back to see if I'm all right. How do I explain that everything is fine.... but it's not? How do I explain the contradictions of PMDD? This isn't the type of conversation you want to have over the phone. It's best that the other person can see the glassiness in your eyes, the exhaustion on your face, the lack of energy and slump of your body.

I fix something to eat (healthy carbs!) and work on a small project that only needs minimal concentration for an hour or so. My friend arrives, and I try to explain what happened. She asks, "What can I do to help?"

The only answer I can come up with is, "Just be nice to me. I'm fragile today. Oh, and you might need to run interference for me at class. I'm not feeling very social right now."

We go to class, and all goes well. I manage to muddle through the social aspects of class. The exercises get the blood circulating, produce the necessary boost in feel-good hormones. By the end of class, which was the absolute last thing I had wanted to go to—at the time I would much rather have crawled back into bed and tried to sleep away my exhaustion—I was feeling 100% again, and had bought myself a couple of PMDD-free hours.

Because in my PMDD-induced confusion and misery, I had **forgotten** what I could do to help myself. Light aerobic exercise. When I'm in the throes of a PMDD episode, and the last thing I want to do is get up and move, *that's the very thing I need to do.* A simple walk is all it takes. After about 30 minutes, I start to feel better. By 45, I'm back on an even keel. An hour of any kind of light cardio activity and all symptoms are gone...

For about two hours.

So by the time I got home, I was back to being myself again. A totally different person. I was able to make it through the rest of the evening without incident.

But as soon as I opened my eyes the next morning, I felt that heavy wet blanket of depression closing in on me again. The iron band around my head, the irritated eyes, like I've been crying (but I haven't), the mental fuzziness, the sense of exhaustion even before I get out of bed.

There's no denying it this time. It's going to be another PMDD day.

Chapter Eighteen

―――――◆―――――

Why Me?

PMDD and Why Me?

Okay, we've heard enough stories for a while of what it's like to have PMDD. We all know what it is by now, and have plenty of ideas about what to expect. We also know there is not much we can do about it once an episode hits. The best we can hope for is to ride out the storm. So a question I'm sure all of us have asked at one point or another is, *Why Me?*

Today I'm going to look into the possibilities I've uncovered so far. First, however, a little background. When does PMDD happen? And How does PMDD progress?

You don't get it before your first period. Girls, on average, are now getting their first period at age 12 or sooner. Your probability of developing PMDD increases with each hormonal event in your life thereafter: pregnancy, miscarriage, abortion, or birth. (You do not experience PMDD when you are pregnant, because you are not ovulating.) With each new pregnancy, your chances of developing PMDD increase. And unless your PMDD is addressed it will continue to worsen with each hormonal event, becoming increasingly difficult through perimenopause, until it stops when you reach menopause.

But don't start cheering yet…if your PMDD is not addressed before menopause, you run the serious risk of developing Major Depressive Disorder after menopause. The average age of menopause is 51.

So, as I said in chapter seventeen, on average, women have approximately 40 years during which we can experience PMDD. Approximately half of those years will be spent in the PMDD zone, less any time spent pregnant, which opens us up to more than seventeen years of time served in PMDD hell.

Seventeen years is a long time to feel and/or be out of control. Seventeen years is also a long time to be on medication, especially medication that studies now show doesn't work more than half the time.

Listen, nobody knows for sure what causes PMDD. All scientists know is it is a biological event that manifests as emotional symptoms. What does that mean? It means PMDD is caused by something that happens in your body and shows/expresses itself in your moods. The closest science has come to defining what happens is that whatever happens, happens in concert with your menstrual cycle, and involves your hormones. The hormones they have looked at the most are estrogen, progesterone, and now a metabolite of progesterone, called allopregnanolone.

Some schools of thought are convinced it has something to do with the levels of these hormones in your body, and whether they are in the right balance or not. But you can't detect PMDD with a blood test, and every estrogen/progesterone blood test I have taken has shown my levels to be perfectly normal, *even when I was in the middle of a PMDD episode.*

I think the best science has come up with so far is that yes, PMDD does have to do with your hormonal fluctuations, but it's more that something goes awry in your brain when processing these normal and natural hormonal fluctuations in your body.

That's right. Something goes wrong in your *brain.*

No news to us, right? We've known all along something wasn't right with our brains, with our thinking processes, during an episode of PMDD. Why else would we say and do the things we say and do during an episode, but not during the rest of the month?

But I won't go into that right now. For now it's good enough to know there is a biological "something" in our neuro-endocrine system that happens where our brain does not properly process the fluctuating levels of our reproductive hormones during the second half, or luteal phase, of our menstrual cycle. This leads to a disconnect in the brain, like when your vacuum cleaner cord accidentally gets yanked out of a wall outlet, or when your cell phone coverage drops. The result of this disconnect "may" affect the level of serotonin in the brain—serotonin being *just one* of several neuro-transmitters that *in part* govern our moods, and our ability to be happy.

This, however, is a theory—it has never been proven.

Ever.

But the antidepressant manufacturers would have you believe this "serotonin imbalance" theory is fact, and this is the cause of your PMDD, because it then allows them to sell you up to seventeen years or more of the "cure." Then, since your PMDD has not been properly addressed from within, and you have long since passed the stage where you became dependent on your drugs, they can sell you these same drugs to get you through the rest of your natural life.

I once bought into these "hormonal imbalance" and "serotonin imbalance" theories as well. Just like you, I was desperate to find an answer to my PMDD that made sense—and these two theories do make sense.

But that is assuming they are true.

Having read as much as I have on the subject in the past ten years, I have come to believe they are not true, and I am no longer convinced serotonin levels are the sole culprit for PMDD, if they are a culprit at all. In his book, *Prozac Backlash*, published fifteen years ago, on page 201, under the heading *Test Tube Studies of Blenderized Rat Brains*, author Dr. Joseph Glenmullen states, "One cannot measure serotonin levels in the brain of any patient. Nor can one measure serotonin at specific synapses. Synapses are the spark plugs between nerve cells, junctions where they exchange chemical messages, and where drugs are said to work."

He then goes on to say that blood levels of serotonin drawn from the arm of a patient are of little relation to what is going on in our central nervous system, or our brain.

179

So to get around these scientific roadblocks, researchers worked with test tubes containing fragments of smashed rat brains to discover the effect various drugs might have on the human brain.

Keep in mind also that most studies use male rats, because female rats, *due to their swings in hormone levels,* are considered a potential source of unreliable findings.

But back to Dr. Glenmullen. He then says on page 202 of *Prozac Backlash*, "To talk about "selectivity" [as in the case of selective serotonin re-uptake inhibitors, or SSRIs] in regard to smashed brains in test tubes where fragments of dead cells no longer influence one another is irrelevant; to talk about it in regard to living humans is simply folly."

Once I understood how the SSRI antidepressants Prozac, Paxil, Zoloft and Luvox were tested for treating depression, and where this hypothesis of a "serotonin imbalance" came from—I began to have my doubts.

That's not to say serotonin levels have nothing to do with our moods...otherwise why would we crave carbohydrates? Carbs do increase the level of serotonin in our bodies, and therefore "do" improve our moods. The science of it aside, somehow we already know this on an instinctive level. Whenever a person is feeling down—not just women with PMDD—we tend to reach for our favorite comfort foods—which more often than not happen to be loaded with carbohydrates.

Whether the carbs affect more than the serotonin levels in our brains is for someone other than me to determine. Now, temporarily leaving the topic of antidepressants behind, I want to say a few things about nutrition. Both of these subjects are addressed in much more detail in my booklets *PMDD and Antidepressants*, and *PMDD and Nutrition*, but today I want to touch on our almost universal ability to, when stressed, reach for the WRONG kind of carbs.

You know what I'm talking about...the cookies, cakes, donuts, ice cream, chips, crackers, pasta and more. For while they might temporarily do a half-baked job of lifting your mood, the boost is short-lived. Instead what you get is an exhausting rollercoaster ride of mood swings and blood sugar highs and lows throughout the day—because you would have to eat a boatload of these cheap fake food products to sustain any kind of real mental or energy boost. Never mind that eating all this junk food only makes you sicker (think diabetes, heart disease, cancer) and fatter—which in the end does not improve your mood at all.

The bottom line is craving carbs is natural. But not just any carbs will do. Simple, refined carbs (like the ones I named above) are out. What we need are the complex carbohydrates provided by fresh, preferably organic whole foods. Fruits, vegetables, whole grains, etc.

But that is not what we reach for. And since we cannot logically eat enough junk food to keep our brains swirling in serotonin, our doctors prescribe antidepressants to mask the symptoms of our PMDD.

Again, I'm not at all convinced antidepressants, oral contraceptives (and now the long acting reversible contraceptives, aka LARCs, the industry is pushing) are medically necessary to treat PMDD. Not as long as there are safer, more natural-to-your-body ways to accomplish the same.

Think about this: Why would anyone want to take a mind-altering medication *daily* for something that only happens a few days a month? I realize some women's PMDD episodes are longer, but for those that run longer than 7-10 days, I honestly believe there is something more than PMDD going on—most likely an ongoing condition or disorder that has not yet been identified—which grows worse as our periods approach. This, as I mentioned in the Introduction section of this book, is known as *pre-menstrual exacerbation,* or PME, of an underlying condition, and there are countless conditions that qualify.

Which is the *real* reason you need to see a doctor for your PMDD. Not to diagnose the PMDD, but to rule out whatever else may be making the bulk of your days a living hell. PMDD, in and of itself, is not supposed to last more than one week a month. If it does, there is something else going on in your body and you need to get it checked out.

What you don't need is to mask the symptoms with antidepressants and/or contraceptives. What we resist persists, and what we put off dealing with will only come back harder and stronger in the end. We will all have to deal with the consequences of our choices one day, and the tragedy of it is most of us will never connect the two; the worsened symptoms we are having and the drugs we have used to mask them.

Also, antidepressants and birth control come with a host of side effects that can, and in many cases do, make your PMDD symptoms worse. But nobody ever blames the drug. We blame ourselves for not responding to the drug, because somehow our PMDD brain has convinced us we are the only one who isn't responding properly while everybody else is doing fine.

This is also not true. All you have to do is Google the antidepressant or form of birth control prescribed to treat your PMDD along with "side effects" and all sorts of posts will pop up.

So do your research and find out what you are putting into your body. Because the body never lies. The body *will* fight back. Just like your PMDD brain, your body is designed to survive, and will do everything it can to warn you it feels under attack—until your body simply wears out and cannot sustain itself any more.

Most of us don't fall prey to old age, we fall prey to side effects. Each time a new drug is added to our regimen, our body has a whole new set of side effects to cope with. Doctors routinely prescribe new drugs to deal with the side effects of the previous drugs they prescribed. This only compounds the problem and obscures any hope of getting to the root cause of your PMDD.

So think about that, and know there are still a lot of safe, easy, *cheap* things you can do to make your PMDD better. Most do, however, require time and effort. It takes time to make good, healthy meals. It takes time to listen to your body and become aware of what makes you feel better and what makes you feel worse. It takes time to find the right treatment for your particular symptoms. It takes time to sort out what is your PMDD and what is something else, maybe a thyroid problem, or polycystic ovaries for example.

It takes time to make time for you, to take time out for rest and relaxation, and to deal with those messy stresses eating up your hours and days and life. It takes time to get comfortable with your emotions, to accept and even welcome both the good and painful emotions.

It takes time to work on your relationships.

It takes time to quit using whatever crutches you've been using to get through your ten, twenty, thirty or more years of PMDD.

But if they were working, you wouldn't be reading this book.

Think of how many more years or potential periods you still have on your horizon, and how your PMDD and life will only get worse if you don't do something about it.

Do you really want to spend your golden years depressed?

You didn't ask for the hand of cards you were dealt. The best you can do is learn how to play them. The information is out there. The willpower is inside you.

So don't sit around asking, *Why Me?*

Wake up and say, *Not Me. Not Today.*

This is your *Life*. Take control of it. One day at a time. That's all you need to work with. One hour at a time, if that's all you have. Like I said in chapter one, pick one positive thing you can do for yourself, and do it for you and you alone. Do it today. Do the same thing tomorrow. Keep doing it, one moment at a time, until you have it down.

Then pick something else, and start the process all over again. Baby steps are still steps in the right direction.

Chapter Nineteen

———◆———

I Can't Leave it Alone...

Because I care. Anyone the least bit concerned about the side effects of the drugs you are taking needs to read *Are Your Prescriptions Killing You?* by pharmacist consultant Armon B. Neel Jr., and Bill Hogan. Another book I highly recommend is the one mentioned in chapter eighteen, *Prozac Backlash*, by Dr. Joseph Glenmullen. For what is Sarafem but Prozac in pink, and what is fluoxetine but generic Prozac?

Did you know antidepressants do not work *at all* for at least 40% of those with PMDD who take them? Thanks to several meta-analyses of antidepressant studies even this 40% ineffectiveness number has been touted as too low. Other studies are finding that antidepressants don't even work better than a placebo for *depression*—yes, the very thing the SSRIs mentioned in my previous chapter were tested for, using rat brains. So how can these drugs truly work for PMDD, whose hallmark symptom is depression?

Again, why this is, and the answers to similar questions, are addressed in my book, *PMDD and Antidepressants*. This book is about relationships. I only bring up antidepressant failure rates so that when your partner with PMDD goes in desperation to the doctor for help, and comes home with a prescription for either an antidepressant or birth control or both—there's a better than 50/50 chance it won't work...

And your personal hell will only get worse.

So don't blame your partner for "not trying" if this turns out to be the case in your situation. And if you are a woman with PMDD reading this and have tried every antidepressant and/or medical method of birth control under the sun, and it still hasn't helped your PMDD, I want you to know *the fault does not lie with you.*

The fault lies with those who persist in treating us as if we are all the same. The fault lies with those who perform their research on male subjects, and then apply the results to women as well. The fault lies with those who have a product that maybe eases one or a few PMDD symptoms and tout that product as an overall cure for PMDD.

They're selling us dreams, ladies. The scientific hypothesis they use to sell us these dreams has never been proven, and *no one* knows what causes PMDD in the first place.

No one.

No matter what they claim.

Okay, so why treat PMDD with birth control? The Pill and several long acting reversible contraceptives (LARCs) keep you from ovulating, which pretty much everyone agrees by now is the main precipitator of this mysterious shift in hormones that our brains do not process correctly.

But again, using a contraceptive to treat PMDD treats only *some* of the symptoms and not the underlying cause. And birth control medications have their own array of dangerous side effects—including death.

Never mind that some women would rather be dead than suffer from another episode of PMDD. I, for one, am not interested in taking something that could permanently disable (heart attack, stroke, blood clots, liver tumors, vision problems, depression) or kill me when there are so many less drastic options to try.

Tell me, is increasing your chances of suicidal ideation *really* the answer to your monthly suicidal thoughts?

Both antidepressants and hormonal contraceptives can help shift your brain into negative territory within days. It can happen so fast you never see it coming. Antidepressant use in America alone is up 400% percent over the past twenty years. Since the year 2000, overall suicide rates in the USA have increased by over 20 percent. (In the fourteen years prior to that, they had dropped over 20%.)

Think about that one for a while.

That so many doctors would so blindly, perhaps even blithely agree to treat suicidal women with drugs that could increase their chances of success at killing themselves makes no sense to me. Especially when nobody really knows what causes PMDD.

How about what *contributes* to PMDD? Do we know that

yet? The answer is yes, but is also as varied as our symptoms. Contributory factors include weight, lifestyle habits, (such as smoking, drinking, stimulant and drug use), caffeine and sugar consumption, stress, trauma, physical, mental, and sexual abuse, and yes, genetics. PMDD can be inherited.

In that case, you really "can't" help what happens to you when you're in the PMDD zone. Because it's in your genes. And if it is in your genes, you're not going to be able to cure it with any pills or LARCs.

I've said it all along: The best you can hope to do is *manage* your PMDD. And for that you need a body that is as drug free as possible.

So what can you do about your PMDD?

You can address the things that apply to you. I'm not going to touch weight, because there are so many factors that go into a woman being overweight that it's the most difficult of all for us to address. But you *can* quit smoking, you *can* cut down on your drinking, maybe eliminate it altogether. Same goes for caffeine—you *can* cut out caffeine and not die. You *can* cut back and even eliminate sugar in your diet and not die. And please don't make the mistake of thinking sugar substitutes are the answer. If you're determined to go the artificial sweetener route, you'd be better off to keep eating sugar. Raw sugar if you must, but no sugar is the best of all. Sugar feeds your PMDD, and it also feeds cancer.

So think about it, and do what you can.

Exercise – If you're a sedentary soul, you can get more exercise. Two to three 30-minute walks a week will do wonders for your PMDD. But 45 minutes is even better. Work your way up to whatever time you can spare. How can you not spare the time, when your life is at stake?

Rest – get as much as you can, especially during an episode. Learn how to Just Say No. Start small and work your way up. And do it gently. Don't put refusals off until they become a full-fledged snarl.

Nutrition – there's a reason fresh, whole foods are good for you. They're packed with the nutrients your body, *especially your brain,* needs to function properly. You can't get good nutrition from a box any more. It just doesn't happen. And taking high quality pharmaceutical grade supplements (not the cheap ones from your local discount store!) does help, but doesn't by a long shot make up for what you can do to make yourself feel better by eating foods as close to their natural state as possible.

Neither does taking vitamins give you free license to eat poorly and abuse your body. Vitamins are meant to boost your nutritional balance in times of stress, not replace what you lost from not eating right and depleting your body's nutrients when you drink, smoke, and/or take drugs—even common over the counter drugs. That cheap bottle of vitamin X or herbal whatever in your hand? Sure, it might actually come from the source or plant it's supposed to, so that much might be true—but guess what? The FDA doesn't regulate vitamins and supplements. It's buyer beware out there. Those main ingredients listed might come from, say, the leaves of the plant and not the stem—which (in this example) is the part that has the beneficial properties—leaving you with no help at all.

It's not about your health and wellness any more. It's about gaining market share. Know this, and shop carefully.

Chapter Twenty

———◆———

Stress and Women with PMDD

Stress and Women with PMDD

Everybody's always saying, reduce your stress, reduce your stress—but what actually *causes* stress in a woman with PMDD?

Well, trauma, for one. Trauma, (such as a life-threatening accident, war, imprisonment, witnessing or being the victim of a violent crime (rape, murder, domestic violence), abuse of any sort, a death or major upheaval in the family, especially one over which you feel you have no control)—any of these can predispose a woman toward PMDD.

How? Incidents of trauma create neural pathways in the brain that can lead a woman with PMDD to *over-react both physiologically and emotionally to normal everyday stressors* in her life by producing an excess of, among other things her, "fight or flight" hormones. Once this neural pathway has been opened, via trauma, the ruts are established and only get deeper with each new stressor, be it big or small.

To top it off, stress can contribute to further missed connections in the brain.

So which is it? Does stress aggravate your PMDD or does your PMDD stress you out?

The answer is both.

Lucky us.

Other sources of stress that work both ways include:

Addiction

Women with PMDD are more prone to addictive behaviors, including sexual addiction, relationship addiction, drug addiction, nicotine addiction, alcohol abuse, emotional eating and other eating disorders (like binge-eating and bulimia), all of which bring stress into your life.

Substance Abuse

This has to do with the reward/pleasure center of the brain, which by now we all understand does not work right during an episode of PMDD. What you think will bring you pleasure or relief from your weepiness and edginess and anger in fact does not, because your brain is not processing information properly to start with.

As an aside, and this is just one example of how my brain doesn't work right when I am in the PMDD zone... I walk around the track at my local gym. I time myself. On a good, comfortable day, I can do one lap in one minute. Sometimes I can do it in 55 seconds, when I am pushing myself, and sometimes I'm just not feeling up to par and it takes an extra 5 - 10 seconds per lap.

But on an average day, I do one lap in one minute.

When I am PMDD-ing and force myself to go and walk around the track, I feel like I am moving through molasses and every step is a challenge. Imagine my surprise to discover that *according to the second hand of the clock, I am actually moving at my normal pace of one lap per minute.*

PMDD skews your perceptions. Of everything.

This includes what you see, what you hear, what you feel, what you think, and what you reach for to numb your pain. Depressed people in general like to self-medicate and jumpstart the reward/pleasure center of the brain with external substances, both legal and illegal. But the PMDD brain *does not respond properly to these stimulants,* leaving women with PMDD vulnerable to addiction.

Other things that only add to the muddle going on in your brain are unresolved conflicts from the past, destructive behavior patterns, cycles of abuse, day to day stress, relationship issues, and cultural conditioning —all of which can lead to substance abuse in non-PMDD women as well.

So not only do the same things that set other women off set women with PMDD off, but:

1. Our brains do not process the information properly during an episode...which

2. Leads to all sorts of bad choices and drama...which

3. Adds to our level of stress...which

4. Leaves women with PMDD more prone to substance abuse disorders...which

5. Are also, in part, dictated by abnormal brain chemistry.

Did you get all that?

The bottom line is it's a vicious cycle, and no matter which way you look at it, women with PMDD lose.

Adolescent Abuse

More will be explained in my booklet, *PMDD and Abuse*, but for here, briefly, studies have shown that women who have been abused in adolescence are more likely to develop PMDD.

Childhood Abuse

A scientific link has been found between women who were abused as children, and women who develop PMDD. Again, this has to do with the faulty neural pathways developed in times of trauma, affecting the "fight or flight" response in the brain.

Physical Abuse

Physical abuse has the same effect on the brain as trauma. Women in abusive situations are also more prone to anxiety and depression disorders, which add to the burden on the brain.

Sexual Abuse

Studies have shown sexual abuse to be a precursor to both Major Depressive Disorder and PMDD, no doubt through the connection to trauma. A link has been established between sexual abuse, PTSD, elevated thyroid ratios, and PMDD.

Chapter Twenty-One

———◆———

So How Do Our Brains Get Us Into
So Much Trouble?

PMDD and Neural Pathways

The previous chapter was about stressors that can apply to all women. Now I'm going to talk about stressors specific to women with PMDD. I'm going to use words you may or may not have heard before. Like neural pathways. What does that mean? Well, let's look at neural. Neurology. Neurologist. Having to do with nerves. Ever have a pinched nerve or experience nerve pain? Ever say to someone "You're getting on my nerves?" A neural pathway is like a dirt road. The more you use it, the more it gets worn down. If you use it a lot, the road develops ruts. When a road has ruts in it, you can get stuck in the mud.

On the flip side of that, think of a pair of shoes. Nothing better than a pair of shoes you've had so long that they feel totally comfortable.

So we have these neural pathways in our brains. The more we use them, the more they can either develop ruts we get stuck in, or the more comfortable they can become. Sometimes we can get comfortable with things that are not good for us. Like addiction and abuse. But hey, they are familiar. Better the devil I know than the one I don't. So in times of stress, we reach for the familiar. Our brain sort of goes on autopilot and says "I know how to react to this" and sticks with what it knows.

The brain does not distinguish between what is comfortable and what is a rut. Left to its own devices, the brain just takes the path of least resistance. To get a different result, or take a different path, you have to *consciously choose to do so*, and in a sense, give your brain instructions to do something different this time. Because even while the brain reacts automatically, you are still in control of your thoughts—your thoughts are not in control of you.

Hard to believe when you're in the middle of a PMDD episode, but bear with me here.

To take a different path, you have to let your brain know that's what you want to do. It will be hard, because your PMDD brain will fight you, of that there is no doubt. Your brain has been conditioned to doing things a certain way. It's quite content to keep doing things this way.

Basically, you have to re-train your brain.

I'd much rather slip into a comfortable pair of shoes than get stuck in a dirt road rut.

Screaming and yelling and swearing and crying and creating all sorts of drama is sinking into the rut. Taking a deep breath, holding your tongue, going for a walk or into a room by yourself to calm down is breaking in a new pair of shoes. It will feel unfamiliar and tight and pinched at first, but the more you slip into those shoes, the more comfortable they will become.

The more you practice self-control, the more familiar and comfortable it will become. Eventually, you will have created a new rut...one you don't mind being stuck in. One that helps your relationships instead of hurts them, and one that doesn't leave you feeling destroyed every time you get stressed.

We're talking normal stressors here, the stuff ordinary people like you and me have to deal with every day. A meeting with your boss, a new client, or your kid's teacher, a presentation you have to give, just dealing with people in retail or long lines at the grocery store. Traffic jams, flight delays, spilled milk, and crayons on the wall. Practice is how you retrain your brain to deal with that stuff. Women with PMDD have a reputation for being unable to cope with everyday stresses. *But this is because our PMDD brains have been conditioned to over-react to normal everyday stresses.* We have to work hard to get out of those brain ruts and we have to start small. One moment at a time.

Some think of women with PMDD as being weak, but I think the opposite. I think we are strong. Stronger than most. Stronger than dirt. Because we're starting out from deep in our ruts, while everyone else is starting on solid ground. And still we succeed. We get the clients, give the presentations, raise our children, maintain our households, keep our families and homes and businesses afloat, bring home the bacon, create beautiful things, care for our loved ones, and win awards, accolades, and respect DESPITE having a brain that does not function properly.

So never put yourself down for having PMDD. Doing so only creates another rut you have to crawl out of.

Chapter Twenty-Two

———◆———

When Things Get Ugly

PMDD and the Confrontational Relationship

No matter who you are, even if you know what you are dealing with and have the best of intentions, when you have PMDD, you will fail to come through for someone, somewhere, somehow, in some way. It's inevitable.

My PMDD is part of why I work at home. I realized long ago I could never work a full time job outside the home. Going to the same place every day, seeing the same people, and me not being the same from day to day...

They would think I was crazy. Like I thought I was crazy all those years. What do you mean, your brain hurts? You look fine to me. What do you mean, you just can't cope? It's a simple report/phone call/task. What do you mean, you can't stay awake? What's the problem? Why can't you think? Why can't you stay focused? How could you make such a mistake? This isn't like you at all, Liana. What's wrong with you?

I didn't have answers to any of those questions. So I stuck to low-paying part time jobs to make ends meet. I could handle being away from home for 3-5 hour shifts most days.

Now I work at home, don't have to deal with anybody if I don't want to, and only work on the good days. When a bad day comes along, I take time off and pamper myself. I realize most women do not have the freedom to do this...however, I *created* that freedom as a result of understanding my needs regarding PMDD. I've built my home and work life *around* my PMDD.

And I still screw up.

I don't generally have meltdowns. My anger is more cold than that. If I'm having a meltdown, you're safe—the only one in trouble is me. It's when I get very quiet that you need to watch out. Because when I get quiet and PMDD angry I *mean* to cut, I *mean* to hurt, I *mean* to wound. I *mean* to kill your spirit.

I know this behavior is unacceptable, but my PMDD brain Does. Not. Care. I am going to come out on top of this confrontation, real or manufactured, no matter what. It's a fight to the death, not because it really is, but *because that is what my PMDD brain is telling me.*

Just like in addiction, when your brain is telling you you'll die if you don't get another hit, fix, drink, or smoke, a PMDD-ing woman's brain is telling her she is under attack and needs to win this one, or all she is or ever has been and everything she stands for will die. Either that, or it's telling her to flee, which is when your PMDD partner withdraws from the relationship, either physically or mentally/emotionally, and leaves you wondering, "What the hell just happened?"

In the case of withdrawal, she is sinking into a deep depression where nothing matters, nothing at all. Not you, not your relationship, and sometimes not even her own life.

Whatever the circumstances, be it addiction or PMDD, what your brain is telling you is *untrue*—but hey, it's your *brain* sending you these messages, and it's very hard to stand up to your brain. (Try saying "It's hard to stand up to my brain," sometime and see what kind of looks you get.) But it *is* very hard to mentally override the organ that completely runs your body, especially when your emotions are involved. It's so much easier to lash out at the person in front of you instead—to blame *them* for whatever's going wrong in your life.

To blame your own brain would mean you were somehow not quite normal.

Defective, even.

I am telling you this now, while I am in my right mind, so that you can see the difference for yourself. In general I am a very nice, polite, intuitive, talented, intelligent, kind, compassionate, and creative woman. I have a lot going for me. I run a successful business, am an award-winning author and editor, and I make my own hours. I am married to an amazing man. We get along great, and being with him is just so...well...easy. We don't fight...even when my PMDD self is looking for a fight. He refuses to engage.

What he does is listen, and speak quietly.

You don't need to shout to get someone's attention. A quiet

comment said without malice will do just as well...as long as your partner is willing to work with you on the relationship. Maybe a code word or phrase between you will do: I'm feeling fragile today. It's one of *those* days. It's not you, it's my PMDD.

I am committed to my relationship. Willing to do what it takes to make it work in good times and in bad. I am fortunate to have a partner who feels the same. One who is kind, compassionate, caring, generous, and truly supports me in my goals and ambitions.

And yet I can forget all of that in a heartbeat when my PMDD comes around. I can be the most selfish and ungrateful prima donna, pampered princess, and spoiled brat you ever met.

That doesn't make it right. I'm not saying you have to accept that kind of behavior from your partner. There are ways to take the fight out of her with just a few gently spoken words, as long as she is open to communication about her PMDD. But anything you say in a judgmental, condemning, or non-approving way will get you the exact opposite of what you want.

So ladies, if your relationship feels like it's going nowhere, it could be because of this PMDD loop you're on. A loop that won't end unless you consciously stop, take a step back, take time out from your heated emotions, research PMDD, find a way to communicate your true feelings (not your in-the-moment-emotion here-and-gone ones) to your partner *and agree to help each other get through this.*

What a woman with PMDD needs most from her partner when she's feeling ugly and unworthy and unloved is your love and understanding. She wants and needs your emotional support. If she doesn't get it, if she doesn't feel safe enough to be vulnerable around you, if she feels the slightest bit rejected or judged, her "fight or flight" instinct will kick in, and she will turn against you. The reptilian brain does not distinguish between loved ones or enemies. It simply fights to win...

Even when there is nothing to fight about.

Chapter Twenty-Three

———◆———

Tough Love

PMDD and Learning to Just Say No

Okay, I looked through my files for what would be good advice, and found all the stuff we already know: avoid alcohol and smoking and sugar and caffeine, drink lots of water, exercise, eat more vegetables, and get lots of rest.

Bo-ring. Nobody wants to do that. Or to be told to do that—yet again. We'd rather look for that magic formula, that silver bullet, that holy grail of a cure for our PMDD.

And while we're looking, we don't want to have to give up our crutches.

We also don't want to have to make any changes in our lives. Like I said in chapter one, change is hard. It's messy. It's unsettling. It makes us feel all confused and chaotic inside, and we already feel confused and chaotic enough, thank you.

But change is the only thing that's going to work for you, ladies, because what you're doing now obviously isn't working...or you wouldn't be here.

I don't say that to insult you. I say that to give you a starting point. The first step to change is to admit that something isn't working.

So, what in your life isn't working? Take some time to think about it, and yes, the answer, "Nothing in my life is working" is an acceptable answer. It happens to more of us than you'd think. Everybody's just so busy running around pretending their life is working because it looks like everyone else's life (everyone who matters to us, that is) is "working" but ours. God forbid we should be perceived as imperfect or somehow less-than.

Well guess what? Nobody out here has all the answers. Including me. Especially me.

But if I had to limit myself to one pearl of wisdom regarding lessening your symptoms of PMDD, it would be this:

Stop looking for the answer outside yourself.

You're not going to find it in a pill, a supplement, or cream. The best you're going to be able to do with those is *manage* your condition—maybe. True healing comes from within. You know what you have to do, and you know that only *you* can do it—be it something you know you need to give up to feel better, or something you know you need to add to your life to do the same.

Here are some ways to start, off the top of my head:

Don't do anything you don't want to do. Period. (If you

have children under the age of 18, you need to see to their needs—that's *needs,* not *wants*—such as food, shelter, clothing, love, and safety. But beyond that, you don't *owe* anybody anything.)

Say goodbye to guilt. Refuse to let yourself be ruled by it. If someone is manipulating you through guilt, put an end to it once and for all. Refuse to play that game. You deserve better than to live your life that way.

If you don't want to attend that event, party, or family/work/church/school/neighborhood function that stresses you out so much, don't go. You are a grownup and are allowed to make your own choices. You don't have to apologize or explain yourself, either. Just say "I won't be available that day."

If you don't like the way someone is treating you, either stand up for yourself or leave. Nobody is going to rescue you. People will only treat you as badly as you let them treat you, and for as long as you let them.

If you're in an abusive situation, get help. Staying is not healthy for you, or your kids. If your friends and family won't listen, there are strangers who will. It's not like it used to be. There are resources all around to help you. I'm not saying it's easy...it will never be easy...but there are a lot more people willing to help than you think. But no one will help you if you don't take any steps to help yourself.

If you need counseling and think you can't afford it, look harder. Many places offer programs and services on a sliding scale.

Most of our stress comes from letting other people

manipulate us via guilt and shame. So find a way to deal with that. A book I highly recommend on the subject is *Guilt is the Teacher, Love is the Lesson*, by Dr. Joan Borysenko. In it, you will learn how to Just Say No to those who try—and that includes yourself.

"Well, if I don't (insert something optional to go to or do here) I'll look bad (to the committee, my family, the teachers, the other parents, my friends, the neighbors, my co-workers)."

If you find yourself saying that...Don't Go.

If you find yourself saying, "If I don't (do this), I'll let (someone I love) down," then give it some thought. If it's someone whose opinion *you truly care about*, then give it some more thought.

Looking out for yourself and getting rid of guilt will not turn you into a woman without morals. You will still know wrong from right. And when the time comes to make decisions about how to spend your precious time—how to spend the moments of your *Life*—you will be guided by your heart, not your guilt.

Once you start living from the heart, you will automatically start taking care of yourself, because you will love yourself. You can't love anybody else properly until you love yourself. Yes, you can take care of them and do for them and cater to them, but you can't truly LOVE them until you love yourself—and you can't love yourself if you're beating yourself up, or letting others beat you up, mentally, physically, emotionally, or spiritually.

Women with PMDD know about beating ourselves up. We're pros at it. It's time that stopped. I don't care what you've done, or what you think you have done. If God can forgive you, you don't need to worry about anyone else. Doing so places them above God. This includes you. If you can't forgive yourself for something, you're making yourself bigger than God, and I don't want to hear it. You deserve better than that.

So think about it, and once you've gotten rid of the junk in your life, be it spiritual, mental, emotional, or physical, you will finally have some breathing room to concentrate on the positive. See if you can get through a day, just one, without complaining. Okay, try five minutes. What you focus on is what you get. If you focus on the negative in your life, you'll only get more negatives. Try it. Starting now. This very minute. Start paying attention. Negative events spiral. The good news is so do positive ones.

But those spiral upward.

So give being positive a try. Re-frame your so-called failures into successes. I made it until noon without bursting into tears. That's a positive. I didn't scream at anyone for two hours today. That's a positive. I took a nap and was good to myself. That's a positive. I walked for half an hour. That's a positive. I got (some job or project) done. That's a positive. I didn't eat any sugar today. That's a positive.

If the opposite happens, that's okay. But find something *positive* to hang onto as you crawl your way out of that pit.

Focus on what's *good* in your life, not what's bad. What's bad is on its way out the door anyway. You're making room for good and positive people and things to come in and replace them. It's the best way to de-stress your life. Fill it with people and activities that nourish you instead of deplete you. Things that uplift you instead of drag you down. Things that bring you life instead of drain you of it.

Go ahead, make that list. That list about what you like about your life and what you don't. Find something small you can do to get rid of a negative. Just doing this one thing alone makes your life a little more positive.

Double the benefit by adding something small to your day that's positive.

Do this one day at a time, one moment at a time.

Because even if you're taking baby steps—you're moving in the right direction.

Chapter Twenty-Four

———◆———

Preparing Ahead for Your PMDD Episodes

Relationships and PMDD -- Doing Your Part

In chapter thirteen I covered 20 tips for partners who live with women who have PMDD. While it would be ideal if your partner did all of these things, that's still only 50% of the equation. You've got to bring something to the party too. As any relationship book will tell you, it takes two to make a relationship—any relationship—work.

So if you're thinking, "If I just love him enough," or "If I just (do something) enough," it's not going to work—not without you running yourself into the ground. Relationships are full of give and take, and only work well when each partner gives as much as he or she takes. You doing all the giving and them doing all the taking does not work *at all*. Nor does it work the other way around.

Even if you've got the best partner in the world, there are still things you can do to make your PMDD episodes run more smoothly. And if your partner is not supportive—then do it for *you*…because you're worth it.

1. **Chart your symptoms daily.** Use a notebook, calendar, or app. It doesn't have to be elaborate. Just write a few words each day: anxious, crabby, sad, sleepy, achy, bloated, cravings, weepy, snapped at _____. Use this to get in touch with your feelings and your body. Eventually you'll discover patterns of symptoms.

2. **Consult your chart/calendar/app when considering social events, activities, creative or household projects, vacations and such.** Making major decisions comes under this heading, too. Don't set yourself up for failure by taking on something big when you know you won't be feeling up to it. Don't just try to slog through your life the best that you can…be pro-active! And make sure your partner knows what is going on so he or she can help you with extra support.

3. **Learn to recognize when you are symptomatic, and consciously postpone thinking about anything that needs serious thought until you are feeling better.** If you don't, your decisions will be colored by your PMDD, and you may well end up asking yourself, "What the hell was I thinking when I decided to do this?"

4. **If you only take meds during the second half of your cycle and they take a few days to kick in, consider taking them a few days early** so that they have already kicked in on the first day of ovulation. Discuss this with your doctor if

you have any questions. In truth, this second half of your cycle is the only time you should need to take any medication, and in regard to antidepressants, this is how they were originally meant to be prescribed—luteal phase only. If you're having trouble with side effects, check with your doctor to see if intermittent dosage is for you.

5. **If you are highly irritable during your PMDD episodes schedule time to be alone.** Don't feel badly or guilty for needing this and do whatever you can to carve out time for yourself.

6. **If you are prone to depression during this time, schedule time to be around supportive friends**. No sense in going through this alone. Calling a friend or family member over to simply talk in your sweats or PJs helps quite a bit. So does having a good online friend or two.

7. **Shop ahead. Stock the fridge with healthy foods** like leafy greens, fruits, and healthy carbs to boost your energy during this phase. You'll crave junk food and if you already have healthy food on hand you'll be less likely to head for greasy salt, sugar, and fat-laden foods that will only make you feel worse.

8. **Understand that if it is not treated, your PMDD will only get worse.** You could end up with Major Depressive Disorder and who wants that when you know it can be avoided?

9. **Find a doctor who will listen to you.** If the doctor won't listen, change doctors. It's your life at stake here. No one has as much to gain from finding the right treatment for you as you do. So take an active part in your own health and wellness. Don't just do what the doctor says because "The doctor knows best." The doctor knows what the doctor knows, and if the

doctor doesn't know anything about PMDD, you need to find one who does.

10. **Try whatever you need to try to feel better.** If you don't feel better, then stop whatever makes you feel worse, and try something else. This goes for both medical and natural treatments. If medication works for you, go for it. If it doesn't, don't keep hanging in there, thinking it will get better over time. Your doctor is not you, living in your mind and body. Your doctor can't feel what you feel or experience what you experience. Only you can know what works for you and what doesn't. Trust your intuition and inner wisdom on this. If you don't feel like you have any inner wisdom, then work on your PMDD awareness and cultivate some.

11. **Do not let anyone make you feel inadequate because something that works for others is not working for you.** There is nothing wrong with you if this treatment or that treatment doesn't work. All it means is you haven't found the right solution for you yet. PMDD is not a one-size-fits-all disorder.

12. **Move your body.** Fit exercise in—whatever you can, whenever you can. Find a few kinds of exercise you enjoy and mix it up so it doesn't get boring fast. A class here, a walk there, maybe Tai Chi today and Zumba tomorrow. Just put on some music and dance around the house with the kids or by yourself for a song or two. See if that doesn't put some energy in your step. Park your car a few spaces away from the door instead of in the closest spot. Thirty minutes of some sort of mild aerobic activity a day is best, even if it's just cleaning the bathroom or carting laundry up and down the stairs. If you have to start with

five or ten minute increments, then start there. Anything is better than nothing.

13. **It is essential that you get enough rest.** Sleep is when your body re-sets itself and if you don't get enough of the right kind of sleep, your body doesn't have the time it needs to complete its repair job from whatever abuses you subjected it to during the day (aka substance abuse, smoking, stress, overexertion, poor diet). The more sleep you lose, the harder it is for your body to catch up, and you fall further and further behind each day. This in part explains why you are so exhausted.

14. **Eat healthy.** Choose whole foods, as close to their natural state as possible. Avoid alcohol, caffeine, sugar, sugar substitutes, anything made with high fructose corn syrup, white rice and white flour, for starters. Start being aware of what you eat, and as you pour that cup of coffee, know you are contributing to your PMDD, and know that you are choosing to do so. Ask yourself is this candy bar, energy drink, glass of wine, piece of cake worth feeling miserable two weeks from now?

15. **Get yourself some high quality dark chocolate for when the cravings come.** Not that mass-produced stuff that comes in a bag. No matter how good it tastes, it's not going to help you like true chocolate from a chocolate store will. There are plenty online to choose from if your town doesn't have a chocolate store. A bonus is you'll need less of the high quality stuff to feel better, so you might even lose some weight.

16. **If you snap out at someone, stop, apologize, and explain to them that it's not them, it's your PMDD.** Don't let hurt feelings fester, on either side of the relationship. If

they're not open to an explanation of PMDD, just say, "I'm sorry, I'm having a bad day," and leave it at that. Everybody has bad days now and then.

17. **If somebody is trying to bait you, walk away.** Don't let their bad mood or behavior spark yours. Tell them you'll be back or continue this conversation when you're both in a better mood.

18. **Ask for help when you need it.** If you don't have anyone in your life who is willing or capable of doing this, find new friends who will be supportive and encouraging. Even if they're just online. PMDD forums and discussion groups abound. You don't need to go through any of this alone. Go to Facebook and type PMDD in the search box if you don't know where to start. Google PMDD groups. The National Association for PMDD is also available for resources.

19. **Do not let your negative thoughts and feelings get the better of you.** Every day, all day long, our minds run rampant with thoughts. Good ones, bad ones, even strange ones. One way to get a handle on this is to learn how to still your mind. But that takes dedicated time and effort. If you're not at a place in your life where you can take the time out to meditate or practice some form of deep breathing exercises, try simply taking three to five slow, deep breaths when you feel anxious, fearful, frustrated, or irritated. You will be amazed at how this helps to calm you. At the very least, when the negative thoughts come, push them right back out of your mind and refuse to dwell on them. Say to yourself, "That's my PMDD talking, not me," and consciously change the subject.

Remember, (as long as PMDD is your only problem), you

are in control of your mind…your mind is not in control of you (even though it very much feels like it, and even though your PMDD brain is doing its best to hijack your thoughts). You need to refuse to give those negative thoughts any air time, because if you don't, they will loop endlessly through your mind, creating deeper and deeper ruts, until negative thoughts are all you know and you end up with Major Depressive Disorder. This is in part how women with PMDD become suicidal.

If you find yourself in any way in danger of committing suicide, whether it be due to your thoughts, the actions of another, or due to a new medication you are trying, call the National Suicide Prevention Lifeline at 1-800-273-TALK (8255) immediately.

Don't be one of the 15% of women with PMDD who succeed at suicide. We need you here too much.

Chapter Twenty-Five

---◆---

An Open Letter to My Readers

~Be kind, for everyone you meet is fighting a hard battle~

PMDD - They Only See Our Failures

I'm one of the fortunate few. Through years of carefully cultivated self-awareness, I've finally learned how to separate myself from my PMDD. I know that I am not my PMDD. But millions more women are out there, valiantly struggling to get though each day, secretly convinced they are going mad. Hoping, even praying, that one day they will wake up and the nightmare that lives inside their minds will be over.

On the outside these women may seem to be coping—some of them coping brilliantly by all external accounts—but on the inside they are terrified by, and of, this mystifying cycle of emotional instability that hardly anyone understands.

They're also afraid to tell anyone, for fear that those people, too, will think they are crazy.

Or worse, they've *tried* to tell others—friends, family, medical professionals—and have been discounted, dismissed, or simply not believed. Perhaps the symptoms of PMDD have crashed over their internal walls and manifested themselves, and those they spend the most time with and/or are closest to have already deemed them as somehow defective. She's a moody one all right, sweetness and light one minute, a raving bitch the next. What gives? What's wrong with her? How can anyone be so freaking out of control?

Women the world over are no stranger to physical discomfort. We can be feeling like something the dog dragged in three days ago and still meet our commitments, care for our families, run households and offices and companies and governments, head up foundations, give speeches, present or accept awards, create beautiful works of art, love our partners, and still get dinner on the table in time.

Women are awesome. We are born with the gifts of joy, laughter, insight, intuition, sensitivity, kindness, compassion, creativity, cooperation, and multi-tasking (our biggest downfall, as we routinely take on too much). We have more endurance than men. We have more tolerance for pain, be it physical, mental, spiritual, or emotional. We are passionate in our beliefs, and loyal to those we love—even when that loyalty is far from returned.

If a woman had a broken leg, and was temporarily hobbling

around on crutches, most people would understand if she was a little tired or edgy or weepy during the course of her day. Most people would offer to help, open doors, fetch and carry things for her, run some errands, give her opportunities to rest and refresh herself. Most would give her some leeway to maneuver as she tries to navigate through her suddenly complicated day. At the very least, they would try to be tolerant if her frustration spilled over.

But when our brains are temporarily broken, as in the case of the PMDD phase of our menstrual cycles, there are no boldly visible cues, like a pair of crutches. Sure, the sparkle in our eyes may dim, our heads and hearts and joints may hurt, our handwriting may become stiff and awkward, our reflexes slow and klutzy, but only those closest to us may be able to tell. We might not even notice these things ourselves, if we aren't paying close attention to our bodies.

So silently we slog through our PMDD days, knowing we feel fragile inside, but with no visible way to communicate that to the world—other than our emotions. All through our lives, we've been socialized to believe emotions are bad for everybody but actors and actresses. Real people need to suppress their emotions. Emotions get you in trouble. Emotions are counterproductive. Emotions are messy and scary. Don't make a scene, don't make a fuss, don't get hysterical, and for God's sake, don't ever cry.

People can't handle it when other people cry. Men especially can't handle it when women cry.

Anger is the accepted emotional outlet for men, but there is no acceptable emotional outlet for women. Women are not supposed to get angry. If we get angry, there's something wrong with us—we're being countercultural. Little girls are sugar and spice and everything nice. Women who show anger are frowned upon, called all sorts of derogatory names, dismissed, discounted, deterred, and destroyed, one way or another.

And so most women turn that anger inward, where it becomes depression.

This is what happens to someone who passes for a "normal" woman, mind you. But PMDD doesn't do normal. PMDD lifts the veil on all those suppressed emotions, all those bitten lips and mounting frustrations life throws at us, turns off the biological mechanism that holds all that suppressed emotion back, turns off our impulse control, and flips all our filters to OFF.

PMDD is your steam valve, honey, and like clockwork, once a month it lets loose.

If you're especially unlucky, it happens twice a month, catching you on your ovulation cycle, as well.

And when that happens, we fail. We fail spectacularly. We rant, we rave, we cry and throw things. We break things, too. Dishes and doors, spirits and hearts, hopes and dreams. We say things we don't mean, and hurt the people we love the most.

Why? Because they can't see inside our heads to where the synapses are temporarily not working right, because they can't see that we're fragile inside on those days.

Because they can't see our mind is on crutches.

And for that, people call us crazy.

We're not crazy. We're pre-menstrual. It's the cycle of life, and it's been around as long as humans have.

You are not your PMDD. It might take up a huge chunk of your life, especially since you probably spend your non-PMDD days trying to make up for all the mistakes you made while fighting off your PMDD brain, but really, who let who down?

Think about it. If you were on crutches, wouldn't the people in your life treat you with more care and concern?

Then why not when PMDD temporarily sidelines you?

You are not your PMDD. It's something you have to deal with, like you would if you broke your leg, but *it does not define you.* No one who doesn't have PMDD has a clue about how much energy and effort we expend in trying NOT to blow up, NOT to burst into tears, NOT to ruin the party, the family outing, the meeting, the conference, the trip...

The relationship.

All others see is our failures. But I read the Facebook posts, and I see how hard everyone tries, and my heart goes out to each and every one of you as you describe for the others how you feel it coming on, how you fear it, how you feel the tension building, how you are in the middle of the storm, how you hate all of it...

And how you ache inside as you do your best to deal with the heartbreaking aftermath.

I am here, and I understand. Because while I have a better handle than most on my PMDD, can even separate it out and still get my work done when my PMDD brain is acting up the most, I know all too well how much energy that takes, and how drained you can feel at the end of the day.

And even when I make it through 90% of the day without

weeping or snapping or snarling at someone, even when I've spent the day protecting others from myself and my moods, moods I have as much control over as I would an eye blink, even when I've done everything I can to make sure I don't ruin their day…

There's always the chance the dam will break.

And that is all they see.

You are not your PMDD. Never let anyone define you by your failures. It's not right, it's not fair, and you wouldn't do it to them.

Take care, and know you are doing the best you can with what you have to work with. I know this, and you need to know it too. Just open chapter one again and start where you are. Right here and right now, in this time and place and moment.

That's all anyone can ask of any of us.